TRANSESOPHAGEAL ECHOCARDIOGRAPHY: BASIC PRINCIPLES AND CLINICAL APPLICATIONS

TRANSESOPHAGEAL ECHOCARDIOGRAPHY: BASIC PRINCIPLES AND CLINICAL APPLICATIONS

Arthur J. Labovitz, M.D.
Professor of Medicine
Saint Louis University
St. Louis, Missouri

Anthony C. Pearson, M.D.
Associate Professor of Medicine
The Ohio State University
Columbus, Ohio

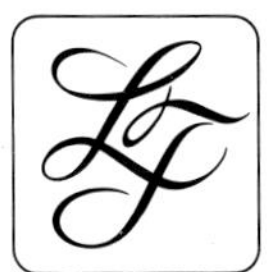
1993

Lea & Febiger

Philadelphia, London

Lea & Febiger
200 Chester Field Parkway
Malvern, Pennsylvania 19355-9725
U.S.A.
(215) 251-2230

Executive Editor: R. Kenneth Bussy
Project Editor: Frances M. Klass

Library of Congress Cataloging-in-Publication Data

Labovitz, Arthur.
 Transesophageal echocardiography: basic principles and clinical applications / by Arthur J. Labovitz, Anthony C. Pearson.
   p.   cm.
 Includes index.
 ISBN 0-8121-1578-3
 1. Transesophageal echocardiography.   I. Pearson, Anthony C.
II. Title.
 [DNLM: 1. Echocardiography—methods.   2. Heart Diseases—
diagnosis.   WG 141 L125t]
 RC683.5.T83L33   1992
 616.1'207543—dc20
 DNLM/DLC
 for Library of Congress   92-10296
                                                               CIP

PRINTED IN THE UNITED STATES OF AMERICA

Print number: 5   4   3   2   1

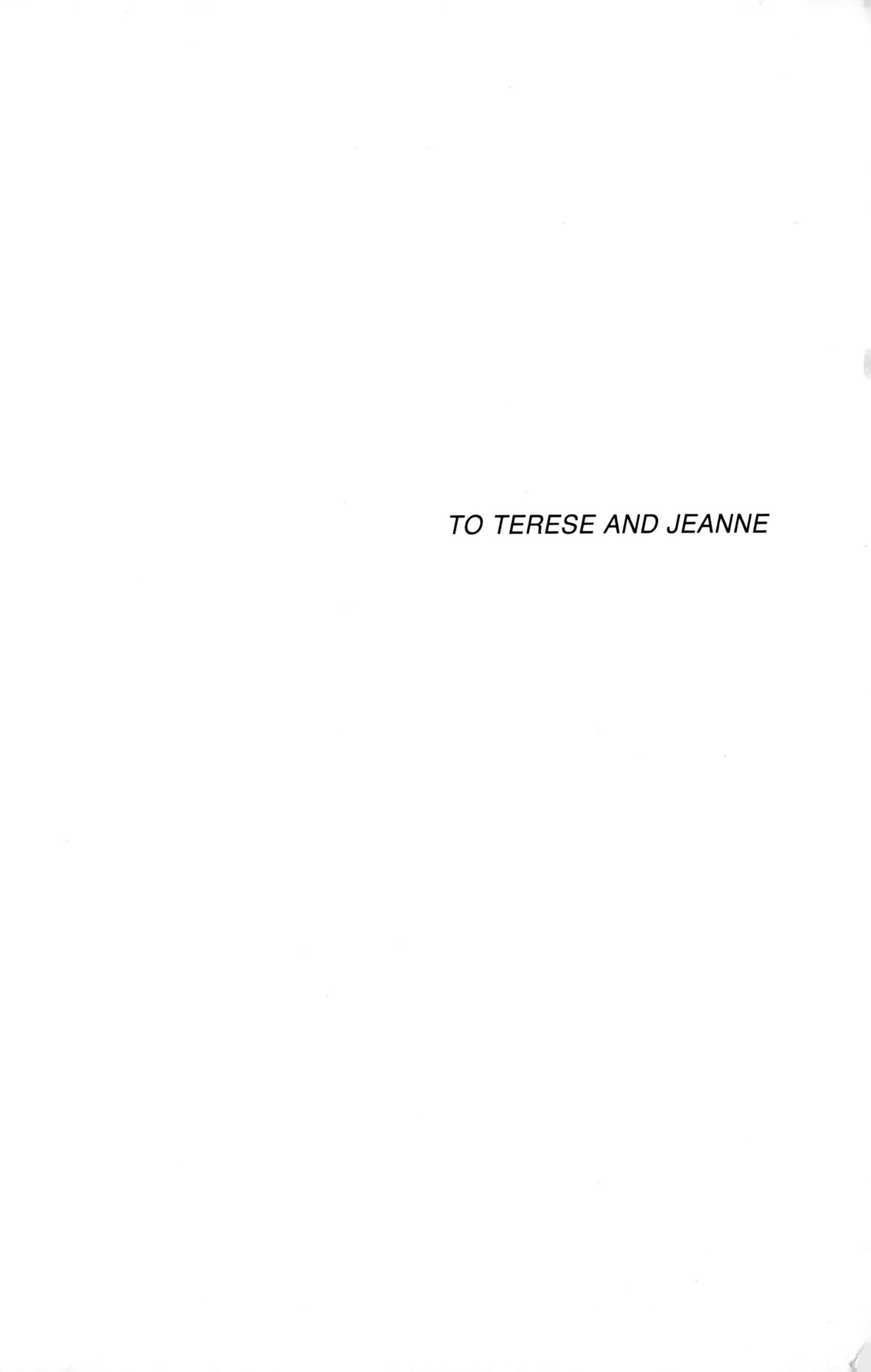

TO TERESE AND JEANNE

Preface

Cardiac ultrasonography has become the cornerstone in the noninvasive diagnostic evaluation of patients with suspected cardiovascular disease. Conventional imaging M-mode and two-dimensional echocardiographic examination provides the clinician with useful information concerning cardiovascular structure and function in a fashion unobtainable by other noninvasive imaging modalities. Conventional pulsed, continuous wave, and color flow Doppler, likewise, have enabled noninvasive hemodynamic measurements obtainable only by cardiac catheterization slightly more than a decade ago. In certain patients, however, acoustic impedance introduced by obesity, chronic lung disease, or a variety of other factors may limit the information obtained. Likewise, certain areas of the heart and great vessels remain inaccessible to imaging from standard transthoracic windows.

The development of imaging the heart and great vessels from a transducer placed in the esophagus has, to a large extent, eliminated these limitations. Proximity of the transducer to the heart and great vessels and lack of acoustic impedance allows acquisition of high-resolution images of cardiac structures. Although the technology has been available for slightly over a decade, relatively recent advances in this technology stimulated clinical application of transesophageal echocardiography in the clinical setting only a few years ago. During these past few years, transesophageal echocardiographic imaging has emerged as a valuable tool for the clinician in evaluating patients with a variety of cardiac abnormalities.

Transesophageal echocardiographic examination is now routinely performed in patients with suspected endocarditis, aortic dissection, and mitral prosthetic dysfunction and in patients with suspected cardiac source of embolus. In addition, transesophageal echocardiography has provided immediate assessment of mitral valve repair in the operating room and is a valuable tool in the assessment of patients in the intensive care unit, particularly when conventional transthoracic studies are technically inadequate.

As the list of potential applications for this procedure grows, so has the number of physicians performing and interpreting transesophageal echocardiographic examinations. The purpose of this book, therefore, is to provide a basic introduction to the use of this technique in a variety of clinical settings as well as a discussion of the pathologic states in which transesophageal echocardiography has been shown to be clinically useful. Practical information concerning setting up a laboratory, description of the normal examination, and an historical perspective in the development of this technique can also be found in the text. Examples of commonly encountered pathology as well as key references are included as well.

We are, of course, grateful to all those who have contributed to this book, including our colleagues, nurses, and technicians. We are particularly grateful to Dianne Reid and Teresa Henderson for their assistance in the preparation of this manuscript. We would also like to give special thanks to Dr. Ramon Castello, Michele Ploesser, Nancy Rickmeyer, Jill Murtiff, and Robyn Dozier for providing many of the illustrations found in the book.

<table>
<tr><td>St. Louis, Missouri</td><td style="text-align:right">Arthur J. Labovitz</td></tr>
<tr><td>Columbus, Ohio</td><td style="text-align:right">Anthony C. Pearson</td></tr>
</table>

Contents

1

Historical Perspectives and Technical Considerations

Two-dimensional echocardiography has in the last 10 years become an integral part of the evaluation of almost all cardiovascular disorders, ranging from coronary artery disease to valvular disease to congenital disorders. With the advent of Doppler echocardiography, and most recently color flow Doppler, the scope and power of ultrasonography in the diagnosis of cardiac pathology have become even greater.

One limitation, however, has continued to linger despite dramatically improved two-dimensional image quality and resolution over the years. The *Achilles heel* of ultrasonography is the poor image quality obtained in patients with obesity, chronic obstructive lung disease, and chest deformities as a result of ultrasound attenuation by air, fat, and ribs. The chest wall performs admirably as a window on the heart in the vast majority of studies (85% in our experience), however, there will always be cases in which this window is simply inadequate.

Alternate windows by which to use ultrasonography to image the heart have been explored by ultrasonographers for over 30 years. In 1960, a single-element ultrasound crystal was introduced into the jugular vein of a dog and the returning echoes scanned on an oscilloscope screen. The intravascular approach to ultrasound imaging has in recent years proved to be tremendously exciting. Its main uses, we believe, will be in the assessment of coronary and other artery vessel wall characteristics.

The second window on the heart, which is the topic of this text, is the esophagus. The esophagus is the portion of the digestive tract that lies between the pharynx and the stomach. It is a highly muscular tube with an average diameter of 2 cm and a length (from the cricoid cartilage to the diaphragm) of 25 cm. The esophagus lies behind the trachea in the neck and passes behind and to the right of the arch of the aorta as

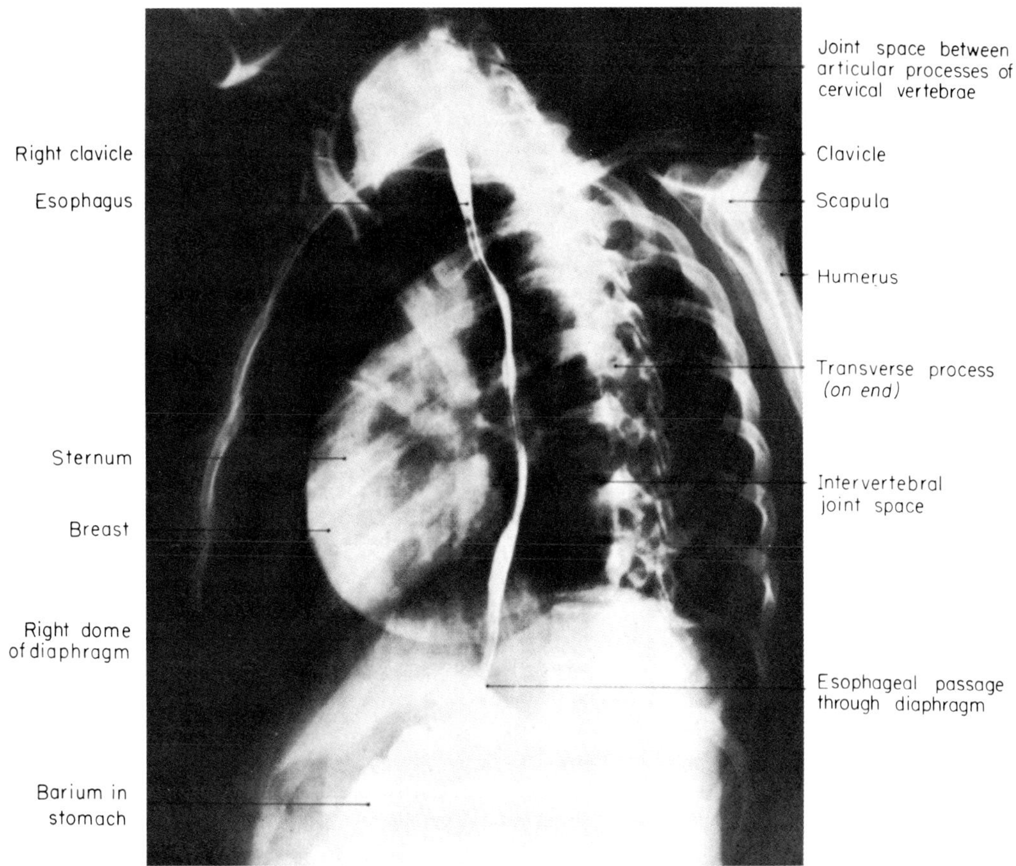

FIGURE 1-1. Barium swallow demonstrating path of esophagus and thorax with a close apposition to cardiac and aortic structures. (From Woodburne, R.T.: Essentials of Human Anatomy. 5th ed. Oxford, Oxford University Press, 1973.)

it enters the thorax. It then descends in the posterior mediastinum along the right side of the thoracic aorta. Below the left mainstem bronchus, the esophagus is contiguous with the posterior aspect of the pericardium (Fig. 1-1). This propinquity explains the excellent images obtained when an ultrasound probe is placed in the esophagus and the heart is examined; beyond the anterior wall of the esophagus, the pericardium, and the posterior wall of the left atrium, there are no interposed structures. Imaging of the aortic arch and descending aorta is similarly unimpeded by lungs or chest wall structures.

Thus positioning of an ultrasound probe in the esophagus clearly allows superior images of the heart. The lack of interposed chest wall structures, including bone, lung, and fat, significantly reduces ultrasound attenuation, allowing the use of high-frequency probes. The high-frequency probe allows greater tissue resolution. The location of the esophagus posterior to the heart is complementary to the precordial window, and the posterior portions of the heart, including pulmonary

TABLE 1-1. Advantages and Disadvantages of TEE

Advantages
- Examinations unimpeded by chest wall, lung
- High frequency—superior resolution
- Near field imaging
- Posterior cardiac structures imaged best

Disadvantages
- Semi-invasive
- Patient comfort, tolerance
- Requires physician and technician or nurse
- Expense
- Limited window/planes*
- Lack of continuous wave Doppler*

* These disadvantages have been eliminated by the new generation of probes.

veins, left atrial appendage, and atrial septum, which are not always well visualized by surface echo, are seen particularly well by transesophageal echocardiography (TEE) (Table 1-1).

Historical Aspects

Although clinical application of TEE is recent, transesophageal application of ultrasonography to assess cardiac function was first reported in 1971 (Table 1-2). In that year, Side and Gosling obtained continuous wave Doppler velocity measurements in the thoracic aorta by mounting a dual-element transducer on a standard gastroscope. The first transesophageal imaging was reported by Frazin et al. in 1976. These investigators coupled a single-element transducer to an ultrasound machine by a cable to obtain M-mode recordings of the aorta and left atrium.

In 1980, Hisanaga et al. first reported two-dimensional transesophageal imaging using a single rotating element enclosed in an inflatable oil bag to secure contact with the esophageal wall. The transducer hous-

TABLE 1-2. Historical Time Table for TEE

Investigator	Year	Event
Side and Gosling	1971	Continuous wave
Frazin	1976	M-mode
Hisanaga	1980	2-dimensional—mechanical
DiMagno	1980	Electronic scanning
Schluter	1982	Phased array cardiac scanning
Schluter	1987	Color Doppler

ing was fixed to the tip of a gastroscope-like shaft, which allowed no manipulation of beam direction, and the oil bag and vibration of the transducer caused patient discomfort.

The introduction of electronic scanners to a transesophageal transducer was first reported by DiMagno et al. in 1980. They used a 10-MHz linear array for scanning of small organs in the gastrointestinal tract.

At the University of Hamburg in Germany, the first transesophageal electronic phased array scanner was constructed for cardiac scanning. Initially a 2.25-MHz frequency was used, but by 1982 this group was reporting on their results using a 3.5-MHz probe. The transducer array consisted of 32 linearly arranged elements with a center frequency of 3.5 MHz, with a 9-mm aperture and a 90-degree sector for real-time imaging. The transducer system was embedded in soft plastic material with carefully rounded edges to avoid damage to the esophagus and was fitted to the distal end of a commercially available gastroscope. The only rigid part of the endoscope was the outer dimension of the transducer array: 35 mm long, 15 mm wide, and 16 mm thick. Rotation of the gastroscope and transducer angulation were feasible by external control. The scanner was connected to a Varian 3400 R ultrasonic system. These initial examinations were performed only after patients had undergone a barium swallow to rule out a diverticulum of the esophagus. In addition, patients fasted for 8 hours, and 0.5 mg atropine was given 1 hour before the examination to avoid "bradycardia and hypersalivation." The authors recommended 2 months of gastroscopic practice before beginning transesophageal studies. They noted a success rate of 82% in passing the probe and noted no complications.

Around the same time a group at the Thorax Center in Rotterdam, the Netherlands also developed a phased array transducer for esophageal imaging. The first such probe had 24 elements with a central frequency of 3 MHz and an aperture of 10 × 10 mm. With increasing refinement of transducer technology, a 64-element probe with a center frequency of 5.6 MHz was developed.

Application of these probes took different directions in the United States and Europe. European cardiologists began using TEE in awake patients to aid in the diagnosis of a variety of cardiac pathologies. Led by investigators in Germany and the Netherlands, reports appeared on the utility of TEE in the diagnosis and assessment of cardiac masses, atrial septal defects, and aortic pathology. In the United States, on the other hand, TEE probes were used by anesthesiologists for cardiac monitoring intraoperatively. Widespread use of TEE in the United States was limited as a result of the perception of cardiologists that patient discomfort from esophageal intubation outweighed any benefits to be gained by increased imaging sensitivity.

In 1987, a combined imaging/color flow Doppler TEE probe became widely available. Initial experience with this probe indicated tremendous potential for enhancement of cardiac ultrasound diagnosis. Since 1987, there has been an explosion of interest in and reports on TEE worldwide. The initial utility of TEE in cardiac masses, atrial pathology, and aortic pathology has been clearly demonstrated, and additional cardiac areas for TEE application emerge seemingly on a daily basis. In addition, some researchers have reported on TEE for mediastinal diagnostic imaging.

As we view the field of echocardiography in the 1990s, it is almost impossible to conceive of a state-of-the-art echocardiographic laboratory without TEE capabilities. In our laboratories, currently performing over 10,000 surface echocardiographic studies per year, approximately 8% are TEE examinations. Worldwide, over 10,000 TEE examinations have been performed, and we anticipate the number will continue to increase rapidly.

Technical Aspects

The current generation of TEE probes with some notable exceptions is remarkably similar in appearance, despite the presence of at least five different manufacturers marketing the probes. The single-plane probes, manufactured by Hewlett-Packard, Advanced Technology Laboratories, Aloka, General Electric, and Acuson, all feature a 5-MHz transducer housed in a 11-mm × 14-mm distal tip. The transducer is mounted on the end of a 100-cm × 9.8-cm flexible gastroscope. The

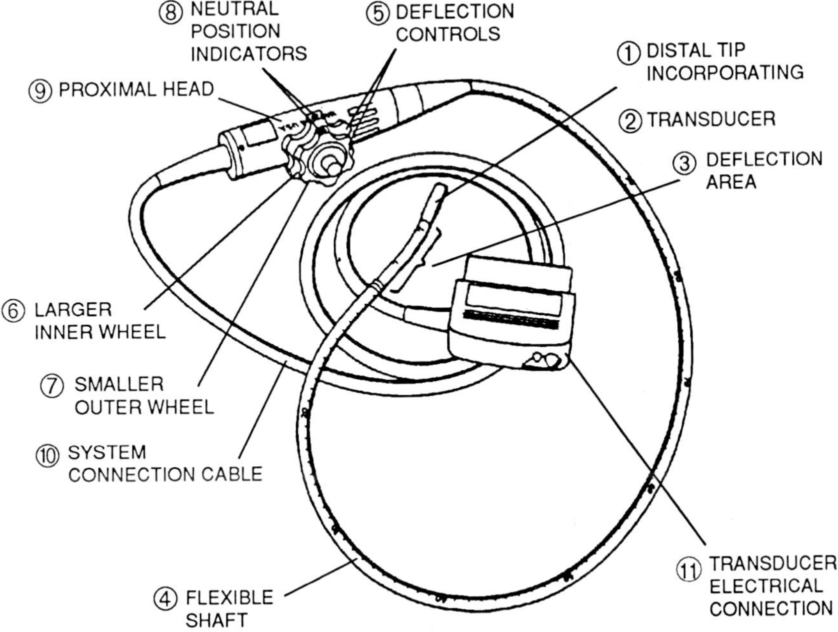

FIGURE 1-2. Graphic depiction of typical single-plane TEE endoscope. (Courtesy of Hewlett-Packard.)

external appearance is remarkably similar because the gastroscopes are all made by Odelph, a small company in the Netherlands. The description that follows is that of the Hewlett-Packard Model 21362A single-plane echoscope, which is the most widely used transesophageal probe (Fig. 1-2).

The distal tip of the gastroscope is 11 mm thick × 14 mm wide and incorporates the imaging transducer. The transducer itself is of a 5-MHz frequency, with 64 elements. There is a 90-degree maximum sector image angle, and the entire transducer is mounted on the distal tip of the gastroscope. The transducer incorporates a thermistor that is sensitive to temperature change at the distal tip and is connected to the flexible shaft of the gastroscope, which is 100 cm long and is labeled in 1-cm increments. The shaft diameter is 9.8 mm. Deflection is controlled by two wheels: a large inner wheel for up/down (anterior/posterior motion) and a smaller outer wheel for left/right motion (Figs. 1-3 and 1-4). Deflection normally is allowed to 90 degrees to the right and to the left and 120 degrees up (anterior) and 90 degrees down (posterior). Because the wheels lie on top of the handle, clockwise rotation of the large inner wheel causes upward (anterior) deflection and counterclockwise rotation causes downward (posterior) deflection.

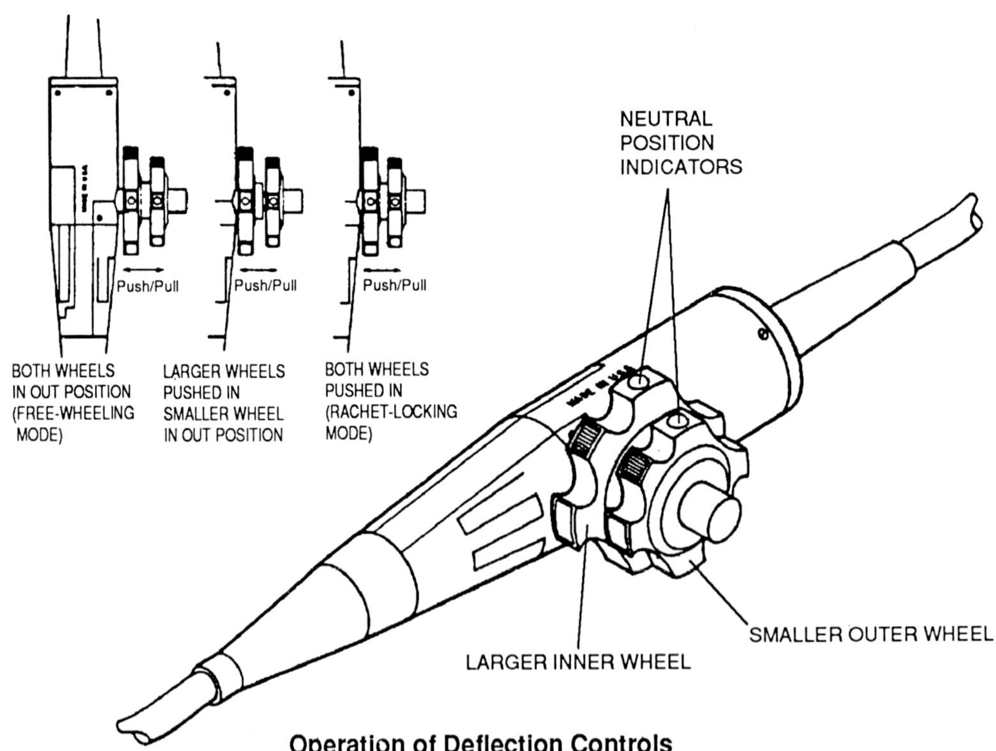

Figure 1-3. Graphic depiction of transesophageal position controllers. (Courtesy of Hewlett-Packard.)

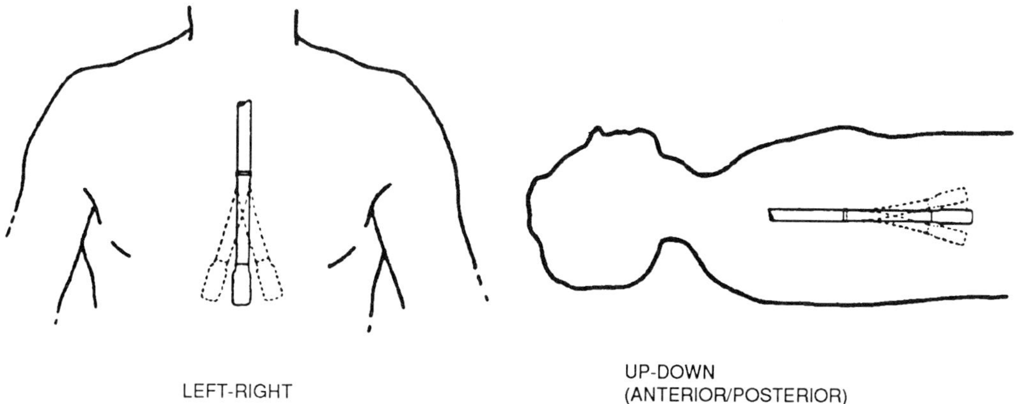

FIGURE 1-4. Motion of the probe tip in the deflection area with left right movement of the outer wheel and rotation of the inner larger wheel. (Courtesy of Hewlett-Packard.)

Clockwise rotation of the smaller outer wheel causes rightward motion, and counterclockwise motion causes leftward motion.

There are neutral position indicators on each of the wheels, which when directly opposite each other, indicate that the tip of the instrument is in the straight or neutral position. The proximal head of the gastroscope provides areas of attachment for deflection controls, flexible shaft, and the system connector cable. The system connector cable is 185 cm long and attaches to the proximal head of the gastroscope. Finally there is an electrical transducer connector that connects the transducer to the ultrasound system similar to other common ultrasound transducers.

Safe Operation of Transesophageal Equipment

Mechanical damage to an echoscope may cause trauma to the patient being examined, including lacerations and possible perforations. Damage that extends to the electrical circuits and transducer connections has the possibility for creating serious electrical hazards for patient, user, and instrument.

Before the initial use of the echoscope and before each subsequent examination, visually observe and palpate the entire surface of the flexible shaft, the distal tip, and the deflection area for frayed insulation, metallic protrusions, kinks, holes, dents, abrasions, burrs, or cracks. If a problem is suspected in the distal portion of the probe, electrical safety checking procedures should be instituted.

Before operation, the deflection controls should be checked and should operate smoothly without binding, and all transducer positions should be ensured. If any irregularity or suboptimal function is noted, the echoscope should not be used. Because involuntary biting of the echoscope by the patient being examined may severely damage the instrument, thus creating potential electrical and mechanical hazards, the use of a bite block is highly recommended during examinations. In addition, the bite block may prevent inadvertent damage to the patient's teeth. Even in patients undergoing general anesthesia with no apparent muscular tone, the use of the bite block is strongly recommended. In patients with no teeth, the bite block is not needed.

Most manufacturers strongly recommend the use of a latex sheath to cover the distal tip and flexible shaft of the echoscope during TEE examinations. The sheath prevents direct contact of the instrument with the esophageal and gastric mucosa, thereby reducing the possibility of contamination with microorganisms. Common practice, however, has been not to use the latex sheath because of patient intolerance of the sheath. In addition, infectious disease experts and gastroenterologists believe that appropriate use of glutaraldehyde (Cidex) will destroy all pathogenic organisms, including the human immunodeficiency virus and hepatitis B virus.

Use of Deflection Controls

The deflection controls attached to the proximal head of the instrument consist of two wheels that permit the user to position the distal tip in anterior, posterior, and lateral positions. Each of the steering wheels has rachet-locking and free-wheeling modes for either holding or releasing from the various transducer positions. The free-wheeling mode is obtained by pulling up on the two wheels. To prevent tissue damage, it is recommended that the free-wheeling mode be used during insertion, repositioning, or withdrawal of the probe.

Temperature Control at Distal Tip of the Transducer

The thermistor incorporated at the distal tip of the transducer allows detection of overheating. When the distal tip temperatures reach 42.25°C during the patient examination, a warning message, PROBE AUTO COOL, will appear; power will be cut off; and the system will stop scanning. If an unfrozen real-time image is on the screen when the warning message appears, the image will disappear and frozen images will remain frozen. If the warning message, PROBE AUTO COOL, appears during an examination in a patient who is afebrile, it may indicate transducer malfunction. The probe should be removed and any abnormalities corrected.

Cardiac Defibrillation

The potential exists for trauma to the patient during external cardiac defibrillation. Secondary arcing to the internal metal parts of the probe may occur. Although the outer insulating layer of the probe is designed to withstand electrical stress created by defibrillation, a small hole will open a conductive path to grounded metal parts to the probe, potentially allowing secondary arcing and burns in a patient. Although the risk of burns is reduced with the use of an ungrounded defibrillator, it is not eliminated. Therefore before defibrillation, the probe should be disconnected and removed from the system.

Biplane TEE

Recent technologic advances have allowed the development of the *biplane* TEE probe. This area is rapidly evolving, and soon all major manufacturers will have biplane or possibly multiplane TEE probes. As configured by Aloka, the biplane probe has two separate elements (Figs. 1-5 and 1-6) separated by approximately 1 cm. By switching between the transverse and longitudinal oriented transducer, it is possible to perform nonsimultaneous imaging in roughly orthogonal planes.

Preliminary experience indicates that biplane probes add additional information to single-plane probes in several areas. The ability to image in the longitudinal plane holds theoretical advantages in the assessment of aortic dissection and aneurysm, and several investigators have found it superior in identifying entry and exit tears in aortic dissection. Identification of wall motion abnormalities involving the left ventricular inferior and apical walls is facilitated by the biplane probe. Other areas in which the biplane probe is anticipated to add to TEE accuracy include coronary artery assessment, mitral valve (both native and prosthetic) pathology, and assessment of the atrial septum.

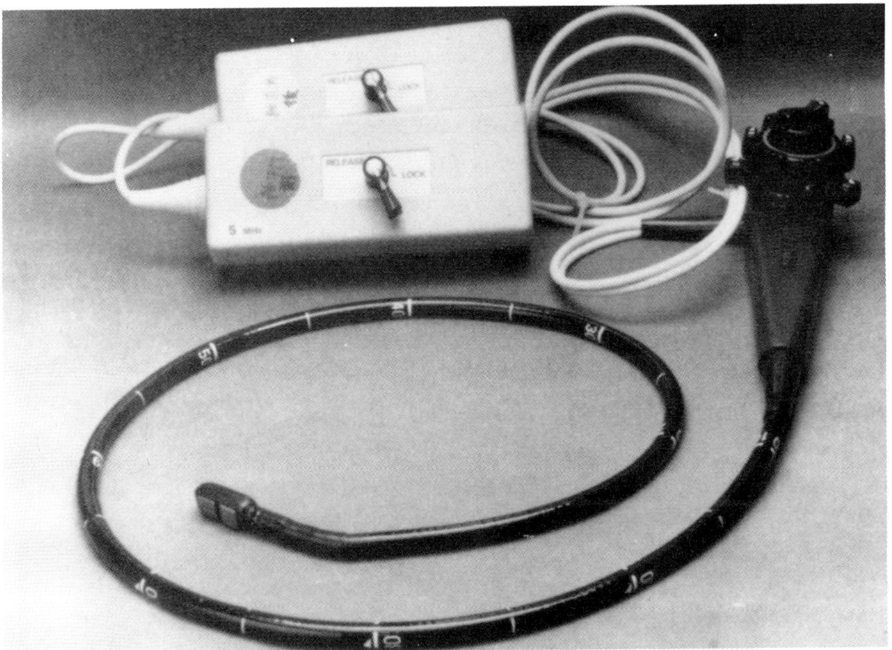

FIGURE 1-5. Aloka biplane probe demonstrating two separate transducer hook-ups. (In R. Omoto et al. Recent technological progress in transesophageal color Doppler flow imaging with special reference to newly developed biplane and pediatric probes. Erbel, R., et al. [eds]: Transesophageal Echocardiography. Berlin, Springer-Verlag, 1989.)

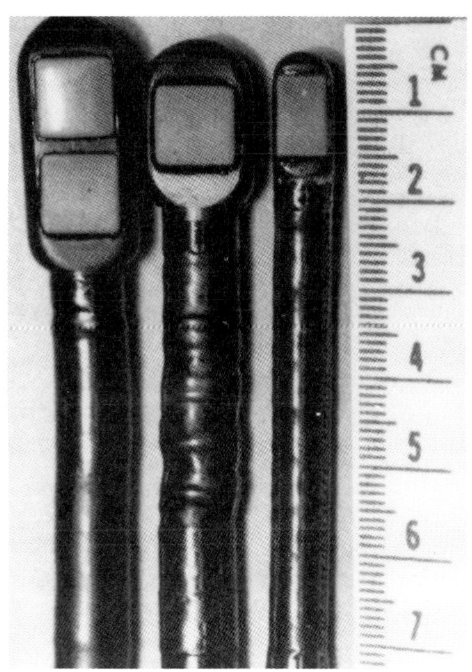

FIGURE 1-6. Three Aloka probes. From left to right biplane, single-plane adult, and single-plane pediatric probe. (In R. Omoto et al. Recent technological progress in transesophageal color Doppler flow imaging with special reference to newly developed biplane and pediatric probes. Erbel, R., et al. [eds.]: Transesophageal Echocardiography. Berlin, Springer-Verlag, 1989.)

Continuous Wave

Although both pulsed Doppler and color flow Doppler are available on most TEE probes, until recently continuous wave Doppler was not. There were no phased array TEE probes with continuous wave Doppler capability clinically available. Vingmed/Interspec at one time marketed the only annular phased array TEE probe for use with its CFM 750 systems. This probe is unique not only in using annular phased array technology with a mechanical transducer but in having continuous wave Doppler capability.

The annular phased array, because it focuses in both the azimuthal and lateral planes, theoretically allows superior resolution. In addition, it is technically feasible to use higher frequencies with this technology, allowing superior axial resolution. Preliminary reports indicate that continuous wave Doppler with these probes can accurately measure pressure gradients when parallel alignment to flow can be assured. The main drawback to the annular phased array probes is the slightly increased size of the probe tip necessary to accommodate the transducer motor. This may result in slightly greater difficulty in probe passage and increased patient discomfort, although no controlled trial has systematically examined this.

Bibliography

Cieszynski, T.: Intracardiac method for the investigation of structure of the heart with the aid of ultrasonics. Arch. Immun. Ter. Dosw., 8:551–557, 1960.

DiMagno, E.P., Buxton, J.L., Regan, P.T., et al.: Ultrasonic endoscope. Lancet, 1:629, 1980.

Frazin, L., Talano, J.V., Stephanides, L., et al.: Esophageal echocardiography. Circulation, 54:102–108, 1976.

Gussenhoven, E.J., Taams, M.A., Roelandt, J.R., et al.: Transesophageal two-dimensional echocardiography: Its role in solving clinical problems. J. Am. Coll. Cardiol., 8:975–979, 1986.

Hanrath, P., Schluter, M., Langenstein, B.A., et al.: Detection of ostium secundum atrial septal defects by transesophageal cross-section echocardiography. Br. Heart J., 49:350–358, 1983.

Hisanaga, K., Hisanaga, A., Hibi, N., et al.: High speed rotating scanner for transesophageal cross-sectional echocardiography. Am. J. Cardiol., 46:837–842, 1980.

Lancee, C.T., de Jong, N., and Bom, N.: Design and construction of an esophageal phased array probe. Med. Prog. Technol., 13:139–148, 1988.

Mohr-Kahaly, S., Erbel, R., Steller, D., et al.: Aortic dissection detected by transesophageal echocardiography. Int. J. Cardiac Imag., 2:31–35, 1986.

Omoto, R.: New trend in transesophageal echocardiographic technology. Use of biplane transesophageal probe. Circulation, 82:1507–1509, 1990.

Omoto, R., Kyo, S., Matsumura, M., et al.: New direction of biplane transesophageal echocardiography with special emphasis on real-time biplane imaging and matrix phased-array biplane transducer. Echocardiography, 7:691–698, 1990.

Omoto, R., Kyo, S., Matsumura, M., et al.: Recent advances in transesophageal echocardiography: Development of biplane and pediatric transesophageal probes. Am. J. Cardiac Imag., 4:207–214, 1990.

Pearson, A.C., and Pasierski, T.: Initial clinical experience with a 48 by 48 element biplane transesophageal probe. Am. Heart. J., 122:559–568, 1991.

Roizen, M.F., Beaupre, P.N., Alpert, R.A., et al.: Monitoring with two-dimensional transesophageal echocardiography: Comparison of myocardial function in patients undergoing supraceliac, suprarenalinfraceliac, or infrarenal aortic occlusion. J. Vasc. Surg., 1:300–305, 1984.

Schluter, M., Langenstein, B.A., Polster, J., et al.: Transesophageal cross-sectional echocardiography with a phased array transducer system—technique and initial clinical results. Br. Heart J., 48:67–72, 1982.

Side, C.D., and Gosling, R.G.: Non-surgical assessment of cardiac function. Nature, 232:335–336, 1971.

Smith, J.S., Cahalan, M.K., Benefiel, D.J., et al.: Intraoperative detection of myocardial ischemia in high-risk patients: Electrocardiography versus two-dimensional transesophageal echocardiography. Circulation, 72:1015–1021, 1985.

2

TEE in the Ambulatory Patient, Setting up a Laboratory, and Indications for Procedure

TEE offers a distinct advantage over standard transthoracic echocardiography by enhancing the image resolution of both the heart and the great vessels as well as providing the ability to visualize areas of the heart inaccessible by conventional echocardiography. This technique has been applied in three major settings: the operating room, the intensive care unit, and the ambulatory procedure room. Figure 2-1 shows the percentage of studies performed in each of these areas. It is clear from these data that the vast majority of studies are performed on the ambulatory inpatient and outpatient.

Procedure Room

Ambulatory TEE should be performed in a procedure room with adequate space for a stretcher, echocardiographic equipment, and personnel directly involved in the performance of the study (Fig. 2-2). The room should be equipped with suction as well as cardiopulmonary resuscitation equipment and oxygen and blood pressure monitoring capabilities. The latter may be performed with automatic, electronic, or manual blood pressure cuffs. In addition, some laboratories routinely perform oximetry by finger devices in patients during the procedure.

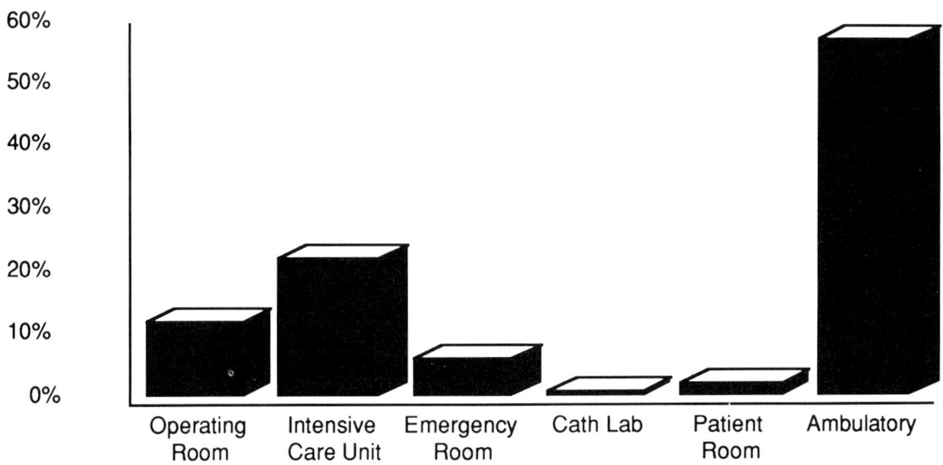

FIGURE 2-1. TEE: St. Louis University experience. Percentage of studies performed in each setting in our first 1000 cases. Note that over 50% of the studies were performed in the procedure room in ambulatory patients.

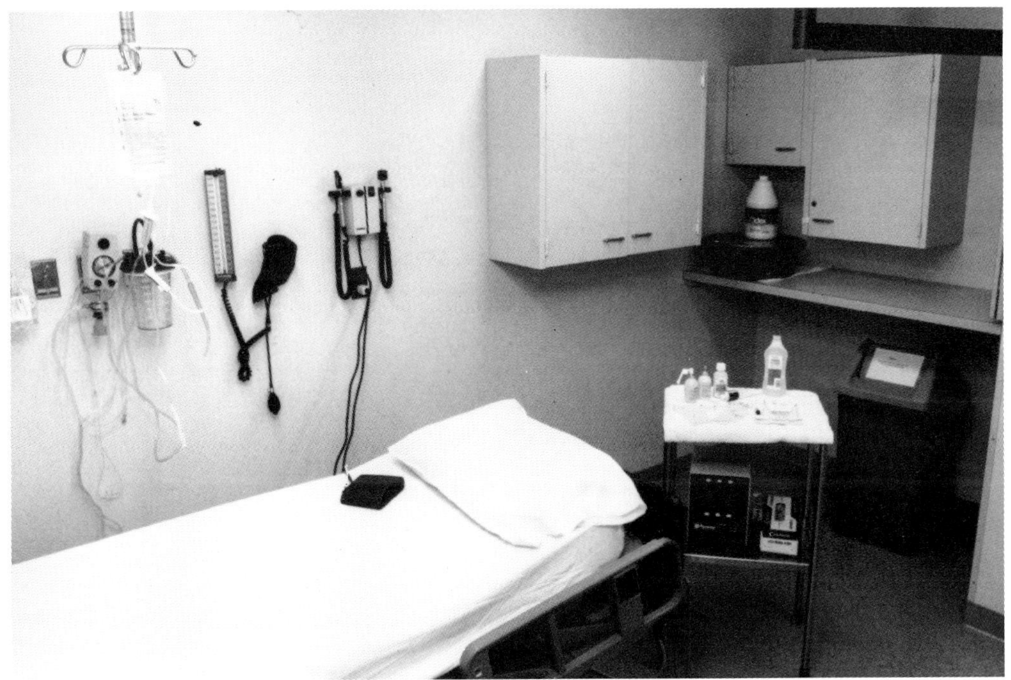

FIGURE 2-2. TEE procedure room. Note the presence of suction equipment, crash cart, oxygen, and both blood pressure and oximetry monitors.

It is also recommended that locked medication compartments be provided for storage of sedative medications and controlled substances. Adequate counter space should be available to allow immersion of the probe in an antiseptic (glutaraldehyde [Cidex]) solution (Fig. 2-3). A sink is useful for the practical aspects of wash-up for materials and personnel (Fig. 2-4). Materials for intravenous infusion should also be available. The endoscopy suites at most modern hospitals are equipped according to these specifications. Depending on volume, however, a dedicated procedure room for TEE or conversion of an examination room in the echocardiography laboratory may be more desirable.

Equipment

Many TEE imaging systems are now commercially available. Each of these systems has its own inherent strengths and limitations. The clinician is encouraged to examine individually those machines in which he or she is interested. Obviously the type of equipment purchased will depend on individual needs. TEE units are available at a variety of prices. Ability to perform satisfactory transthoracic echocardiographic studies is a major consideration. Operator ease of use, portability, and

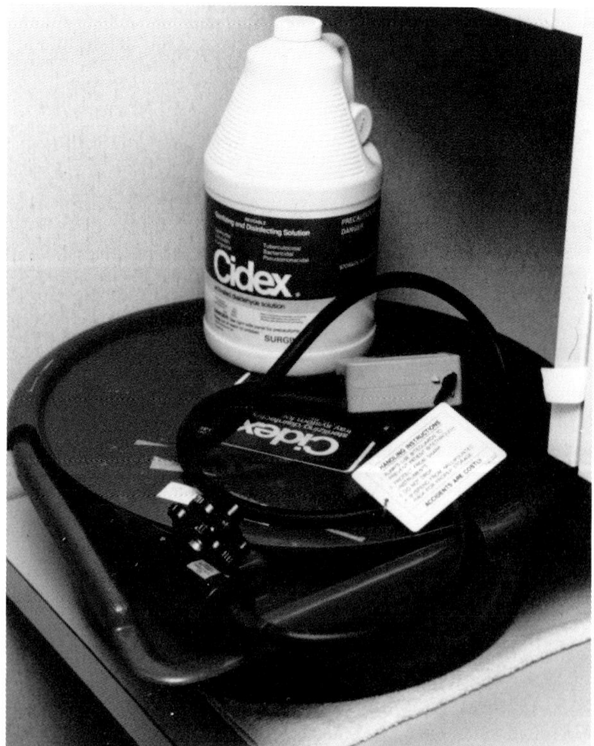

FIGURE 2-3. Probes are placed in Cidex disinfecting solution for at least 10 minutes between procedures.

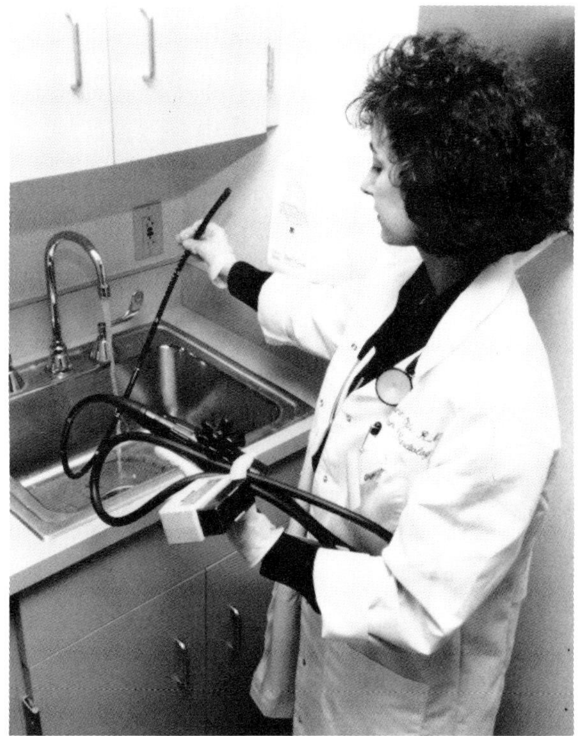

FIGURE 2-4. The probe should be rinsed in tap water after removing from disinfectant solution.

Doppler capabilities are also major considerations. Probe size and individual need for biplane or multiplane capabilities may vary from laboratory to laboratory. Probe size, shape, and durability may vary from machine to machine as well. Adequate space should be allowed in the procedure room for storage of the probe between patients. The probe should be examined for cracks in the casing as well as proper functioning of flexion dials before procedures.

Personnel

Appropriately trained personnel are necessary to perform TEE properly. The cardiologist performing the procedure needs specific training in placement, manipulation, and interpretation of transesophageal studies. Although specific criteria for independent performance of these examinations have not yet been mandated, it is suggested that approximately 20 to 40 transesophageal studies be performed under supervision of an experienced operator (either an experienced cardiologist or gastroenterologist). A nurse, although not mandatory, is recommended as part of the personnel of a well-staffed TEE procedure team. This individual should be adept at the administration of medication, monitoring of vital signs, and attending to patient needs during the procedure, including suction, oxygen administration, and reassurance. Proper history taking and preparation for each procedure are quite helpful in the performance of transesophageal studies. Part of the nurse's job should include assurance that the patient takes nothing by mouth for at least 4 to 6 hours before the procedure, facilitation of the patient's transport to and from the procedure room, and recovery, if necessary, from intravenous sedation following the procedure. In addition, individualized functions such as administration of antibiotic prophylaxis and obtaining prothrombin time values in patients on anticoagulants can be routinely performed by this individual. Finally it is helpful to have an individual adept at the manipulation of the echocardiographic machine while the physician is performing the examination. This is usually best accomplished by a skilled sonographer who can quickly accomplish changes in modality, depth, gain, and compression settings.

Indications for the Procedure

Although the list of applications of TEE continues to grow, there are certain specific conditions in which TEE has been shown to be clinically useful and to provide superior information to transthoracic echocardiography (Fig. 2-5). Each of these specific applications is discussed in greater detail in subsequent chapters.

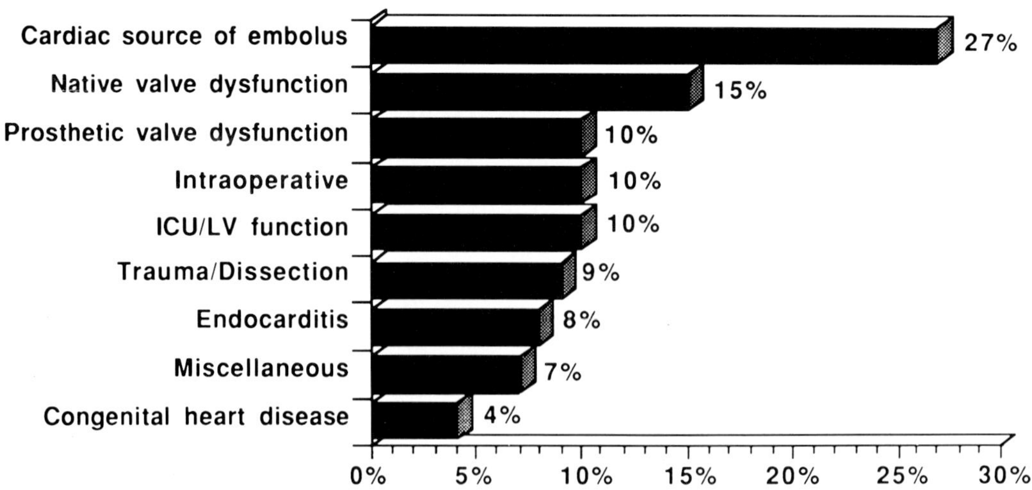

FIGURE 2-5. TEE: St. Louis University experience (1000 cases). Percentage of studies performed for various clinical indications in an active echocardiography laboratory.

Technically Inadequate Study

Because of acoustic impedance secondary to either body habitus or lung disease, information gained from transthoracic echocardiography may be unsatisfactory. TEE performed in these patients is clinically indicated.

Cardiac Source of Embolus

Approximately one in five of all TEEs performed in an active laboratory is performed for this indication. Up to 50% of patients with unexplained cerebral ischemia may have a possible etiology determined by this technique.

Aortic Dissection

Diagnosis of aortic dissection can be made with a very high sensitivity and specificity by TEE. The site of intimal tear and associated cardiac abnormality may be demonstrated.

Mitral Valve Abnormalities

Because of the proximity of the mitral valve and left atrium to the transesophageal probe, anatomic abnormalities of the mitral valve and apparatus can be clearly seen. Quantitation of the severity of mitral insufficiency is also greatly enhanced by this technique.

Prosthetic Valve Dysfunction

Suspected prosthetic valve dysfunction, particularly in the mitral position, is enhanced by TEE. This technique should be used routinely in such patients.

Atrial Pathology

In addition to masses in either the left or the right atrium, atrial septum, and atrial appendages can be explored to a much greater degree by TEE. The presence of intra-atrial shunting through a patent foramen ovale or atrial septal defect is best appreciated by TEE. In addition, the diagnosis of atrial septal aneurysm can be made with a much higher degree of sensitivity by TEE.

Congenital Heart Disease

TEE may provide more detailed information in describing a variety of congenital cardiac abnormalities. Sensitivity of atrial or ventricular septal defects may be enhanced by this technique. Complex lesions and postoperative assessment may also be assessed with greater resolution by TEE.

Endocarditis

The sensitivity in the diagnosis of valvular vegetations as well as diagnosis of complications, including hemodynamic abnormalities (insufficiency) and development of abscess formation, can be better assessed by TEE.

Bibliography

Daniel, W.G., Mugge, A., Eschenbruch, C., Lichtlen, P.R.: Practicability of transesophageal echocardiography in conscious patients. *In* Transesophageal Echocardiography. Edited by R. Erbel, et al. Berlin, Springer-Verlag, 1989, pp 354–358.

Geibel, A., Kasper, W., Behroz, A., et al.: Risk of transesophageal echocardiography in awake patients with cardiac diseases. Am. J. Cardiol., 62:337–339, 1988.

Mitchell, M.M., Sutherland, G.R., Gussenhoven, E.J., et al.: Transesophageal echocardiography. J. Am. Soc. Echo., 1:362–377, 1988.

Pavlides, G.S., Hauser, A.M., Stewart, J.R., et al.: Contribution of transesophageal echocardiography to patient diagnosis and treatment: A prospective analysis. Am. Heart J., 120:910–914, 1990.

Phillips, J.: Transesophageal echocardiography: The cardiac sonographer's role. J. Am. Soc. Echo., 3:73–74, 1989.

Schiller, N.B., Maurer, G., Ritter, S.B., et al.: Transesophageal echocardiography. J. Am. Soc. Echo., 2:354, 1989.

Zabalgoitia, M., Gandhi, D.K., Evans, J., et al.: Transesophageal echocardiography in the awake elderly patient: Its role in the clinical decision-making process. Am. Heart J., 120:1147–1153, 1990.

3

TEE Examination: Procedure and Standard Views

The technique involved in the performance of the TEE examination has evolved over the past several years in the laboratories in which a great many of these studies have been performed. Although there still remains individual variability in the technique from laboratory to laboratory, there are important considerations and standard views that are necessary to understand to perform and interpret these studies successfully.

Procedure

Preparation

The procedure should be explained to the patient before undergoing the study to help alleviate anxiety and inform the patient what to expect. A small booklet with illustrations is sometimes helpful in this regard (Fig. 3-1). Adequate history should be obtained, including specific questions concerning gastrointestinal symptoms and difficulty swallowing. Patients on anticoagulant therapy should have prothrombin time values checked, and the need for antibiotic prophylaxis should be assessed in high-risk patients. Patients should fast for at least 4 to 6 hours before the procedure to decrease the risk of aspiration. Outpatients should have another responsible individual drive them to the hospital. Intravenous access should be obtained, and sedation can be achieved through the administration of midazolam (Versed), diazepam (Valium), meperidine (Demerol), or a combination of these medications (Table 3-1). Failure to intubate the esophagus is most often related to

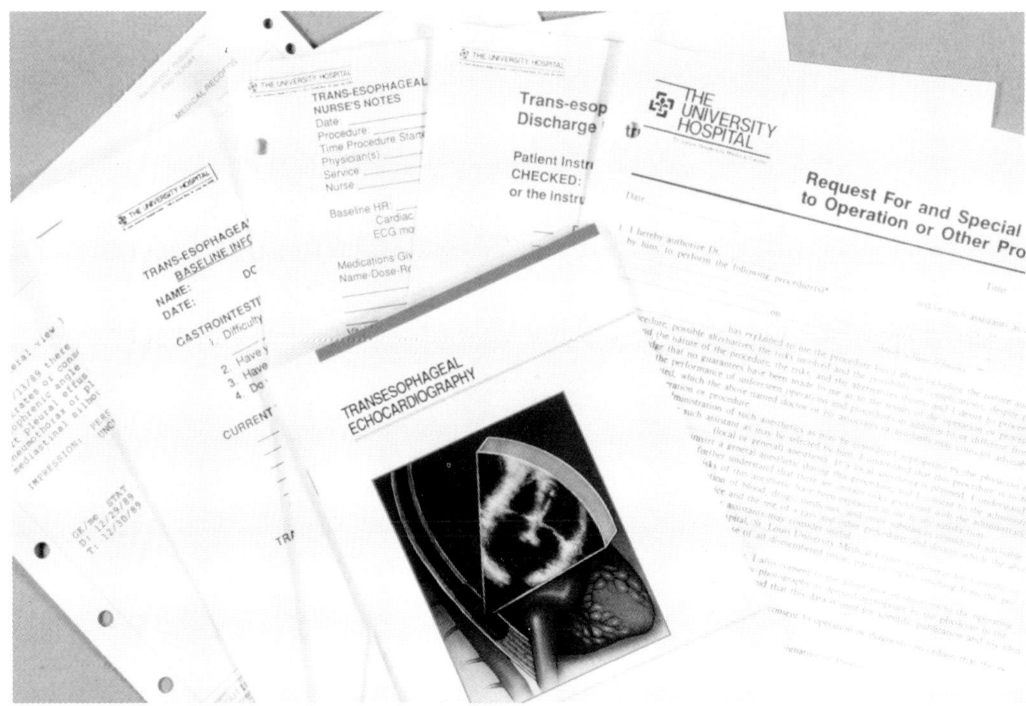

FIGURE 3-1. A patient information booklet (foreground) is useful for patient review before the procedure. Consent form, detailed history, nurses' notes, and other pertinent information associated with the examination are shown in the background.

inadequate sedation and high patient anxiety. The hypopharynx should be anesthetized with topical agents of lidocaine, Cetacaine, or benzocaine base (Fig. 3-2). The procedure should not be attempted until elimination of the gag reflex. Blood pressure should be measured before the administration of intravenous sedation and monitored throughout the procedure. The probe should be examined for cracks in the casing be-

TABLE 3-1. Intravenous Sedation

	Dose	Duration	Advantages	Adverse Effects
Midazolam (Versed)	1–5 mg	30–60 min	Short-acting amnesia	Respiratory depression
Diazepam (Valium)	2.5–10 mg	1–2 hr	Amnesia	Respiratory depression
Meperidine (Demerol)	12.5–50 mg	2–4 hr	Reversible with naloxone (Narcan)	Respiratory depression
Morphine	2–10 mg	1–2 hr	Reversible with Narcan	Respiratory depression

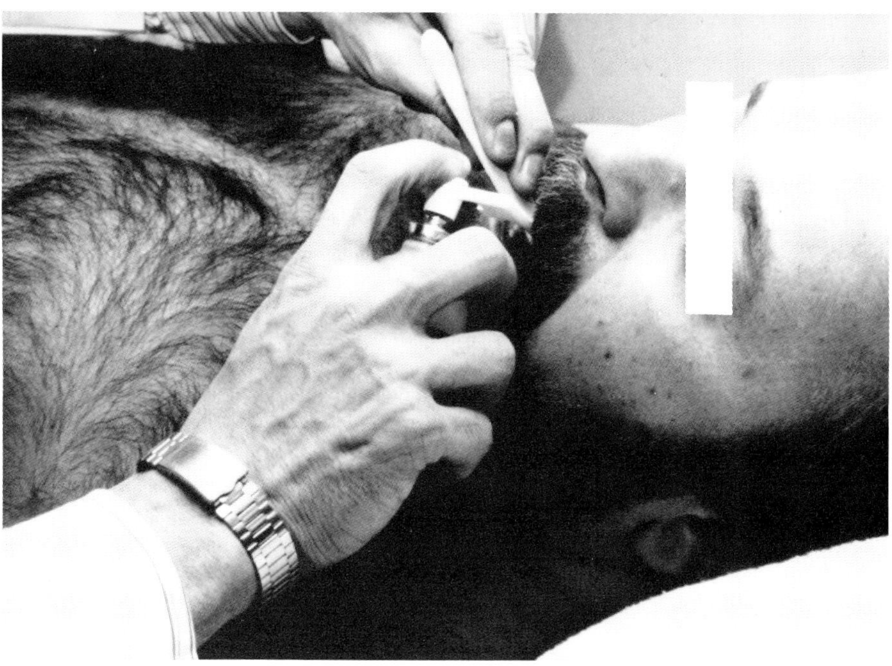

FIGURE 3-2. The hypopharynx often needs to be sprayed several times to obtain adequate topical anesthesia and elimination of the gag reflex.

fore the procedure. Flexion knobs should be checked for proper function.

Esophageal Intubation

The procedure is usually begun with the patient in the left lateral decubitus position to prevent aspiration. The probe is placed in the oropharynx and then advanced into the esophagus as the patient is asked to swallow. The probe may be guided to the midline with the introduction of one or two fingers into the patient's mouth (Fig. 3-3). Alternatively a bite block may be placed before the introduction of the probe, with the probe being advanced blindly into the oropharynx and esophagus. Sometimes flexion of the neck is helpful in advancing the probe into the esophagus. On occasion, a laryngoscope may be useful in visualizing the esophagus in anesthetized patients or those with an endotracheal tube. Once the probe has been introduced into the esophagus, it is advanced to approximately 30 cm from the incisors.

The patient is monitored throughout the procedure, which usually takes between 10 and 30 minutes. Blood pressure and heart rate should be monitored throughout. Suction may be necessary to clear secretions at intervals throughout the procedure. Some laboratories use intravenous glycopyrrolate to reduce secretions. Monitoring of arterial oxygen saturation can be accomplished by finger oximetry in patients with

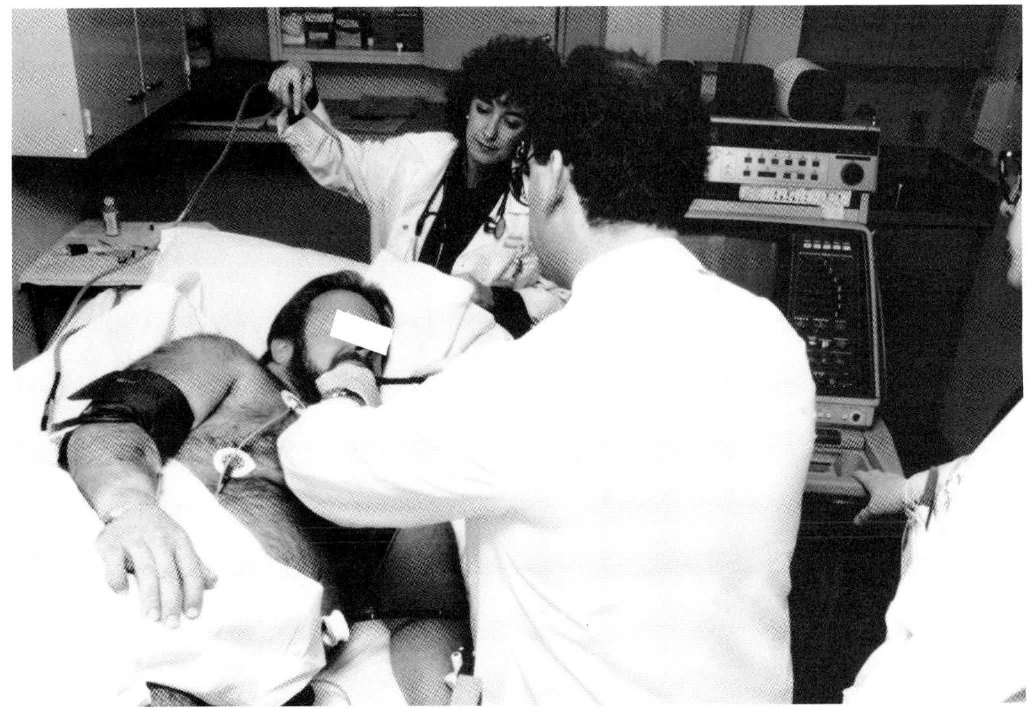

FIGURE 3-3. As the probe is introduced to the proximal esophagus, the patient is asked to swallow and may experience some discomfort at this point. The nurse should be available for suctioning and patient reassurance.

borderline respiratory status. During the procedure, 10 ml of agitated saline may be injected to assess for intercardiac shunting. The probe should not be advanced in a flexed position. The primary goal of the examination is to answer the clinical question for which the test is indicated.

Standard Views: Single Plane

Basal Short Axis View

The basal short axis view (Fig. 3-4) is encountered approximately 25 to 35 cm from the incisors. This view is usually best imaged with some flexion of the transducer tip. At appropriate depth settings, the aorta will occupy the center of the field with the aortic leaflets clearly seen. On the right side of the screen, left atrial appendage and the superior left atrium can be seen (Fig. 3-5) and with additional rotation, the entrance of the left upper pulmonary vein into the atrium (Fig. 3-6). With rotation to the right, the right upper pulmonary vein can be visualized as well as the superior vena cava and the right atrial appendage or superior right atrium. Pulmonary venous flow can be examined extensively by TEE. Left upper pulmonary vein usually provides flow that is most parallel to the interrogating Doppler beam. The normal flow pattern includes forward or antegrade flow occurring during both systole and diastole. Systolic forward flow is frequently biphasic and is

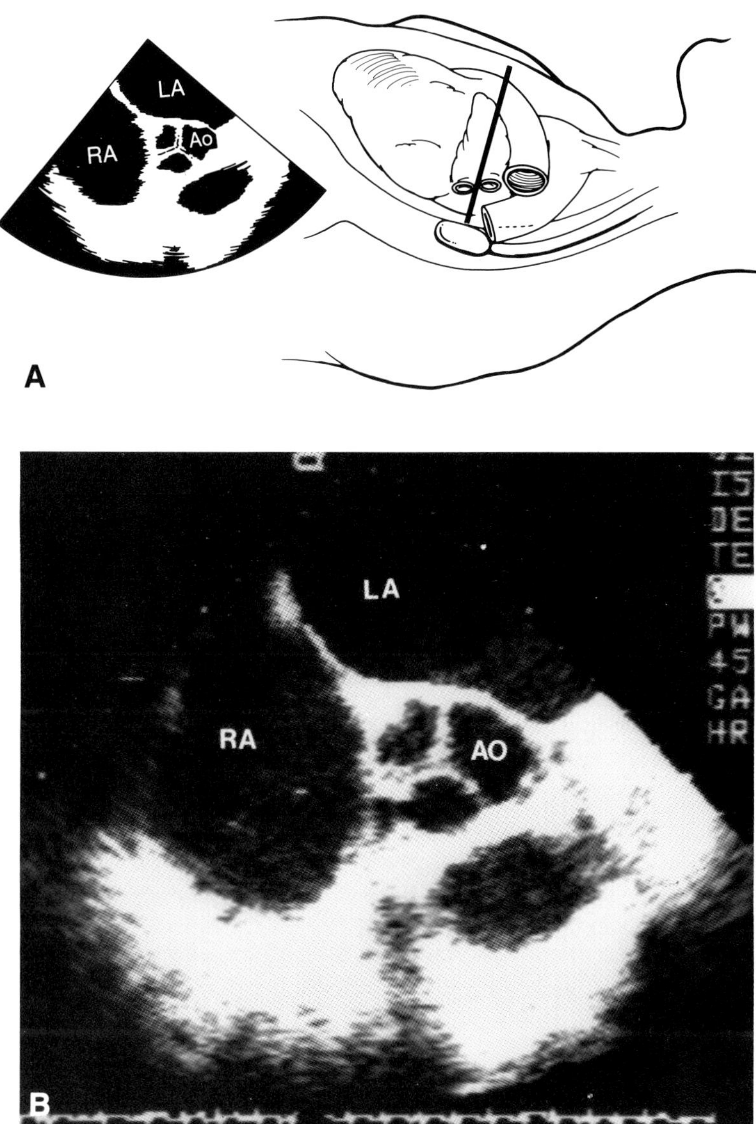

FIGURE 3-4. A. Transesophageal transducer placement with schematic two-dimensional image. B. Actual image at the basal short axis window in the upper esophagus. Note the flexed position of the transducer allows excellent visualization of the left atrium (LA), interatrial septum, right atrium (RA), and trileaflet aortic valve (Ao). The right ventricular outflow tract can be seen in the far field below the aorta.

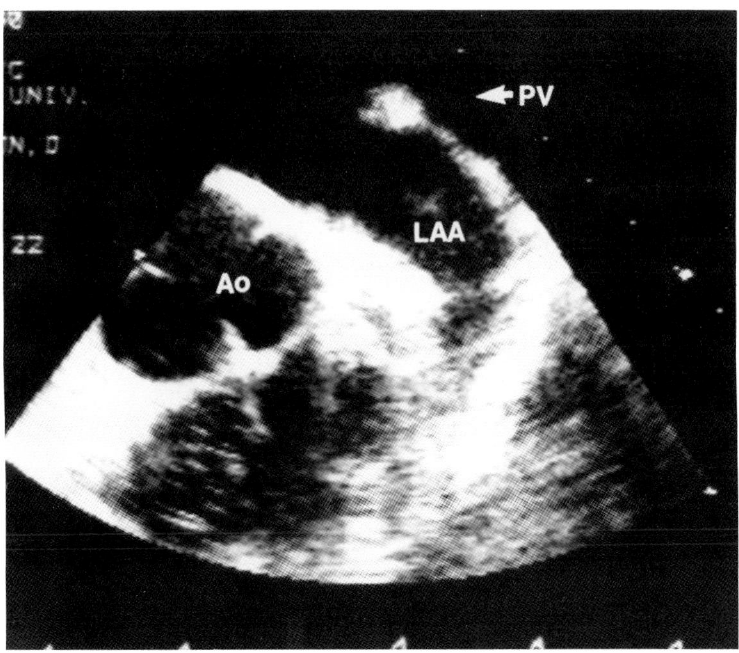

FIGURE 3-5. View slightly above Figure 3-4 demonstrating a triangular-shaped left atrial appendage. Small pectinate muscles can be seen within the appendage. The pulmonary vein is to the right of the screen.

secondary to atrial relaxation as well as ventricular systole. Systolic pulmonary venous flow correlates with cardiac output and stroke volume and is related to the displacement of the mitral valve annulus toward the ventricular apex. Advancing the probe slightly will bring the intra-atrial septum into view. The fossa ovalis is seen as a thin area of the intra-atrial septum. Concentrating on the proximal ascending aorta, slight probe manipulations including advancement, flexion, or both will usually allow visualization of the left coronary artery (Fig. 3-7) occupying a position at approximately 3 o'clock and oftentimes the origin of the proximal right coronary artery at approximately 7 o'clock. Right ventricular outflow is seen at the bottom of the screen. Withdrawing and flexing the probe will often allow visualization of the main pulmonary artery and its bifurcation (Fig. 3-8).

Four-Chamber View

Slight advancement of the probe to a depth of 30 to 35 cm should allow visualization of the four-chamber view (Fig. 3-9). This is usually best accomplished by allowing the probe tip to assume a neutral or even somewhat retroflexed configuration. The left and right atria are now seen at the top of the screen with the ventricular apex at the bottom. The interatrial septum can be clearly visualized as well as both the mitral and the tricuspid valves. Slight transducer flexion and rotation

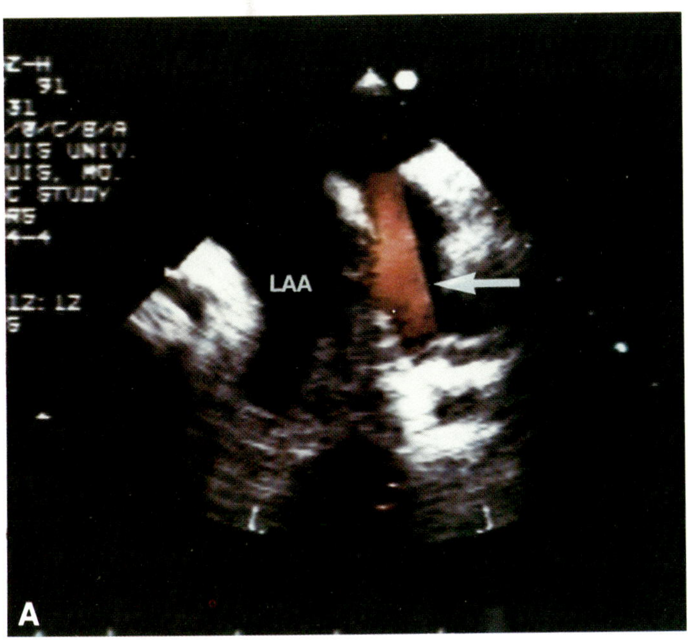

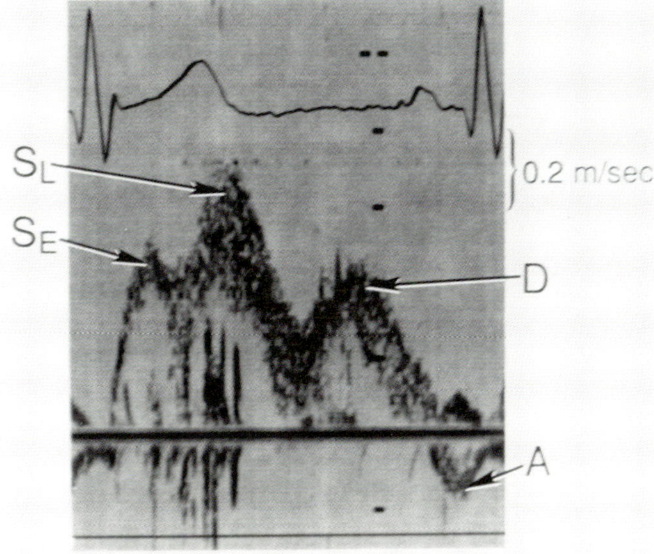

FIGURE 3-6. A. TEE view in upper esophagus demonstrating flow in the left upper pulmonary view (*arrow*). LAA = left atrial appendage. B. Typical pulmonary venous flow tracing exhibiting the biphasic systolic components (S_L, S_E), a diastolic wave (D), and atrial systole (A).

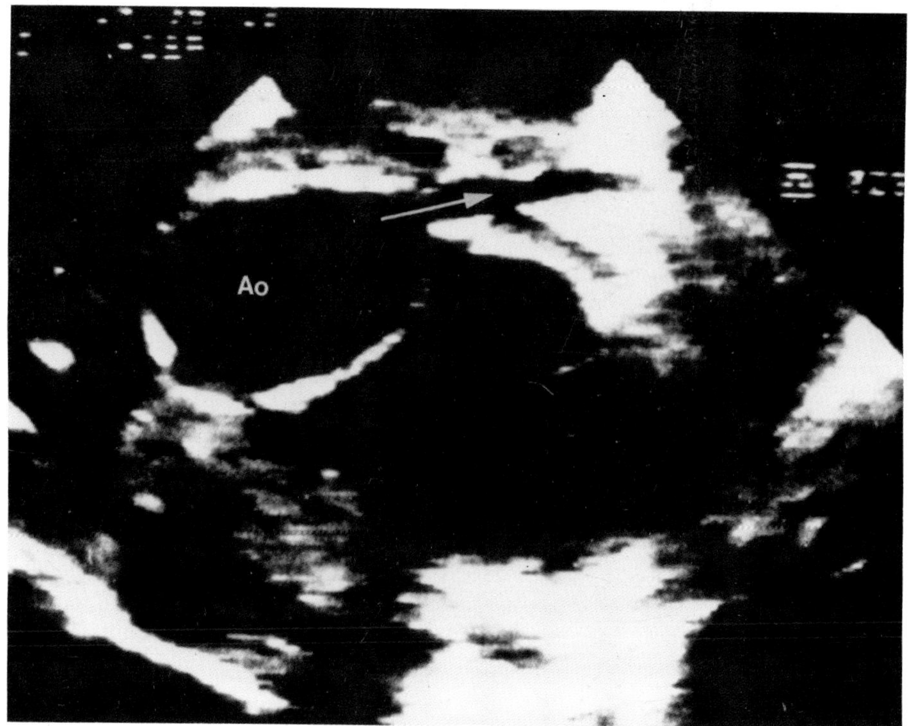

FIGURE 3-7. Origin of the left main coronary artery (*arrow*) from the aortic root (Ao). Note the bifurcation of the left coronary system and visualization of the proximal circumflex (upper) and left anterior descending coronary artery.

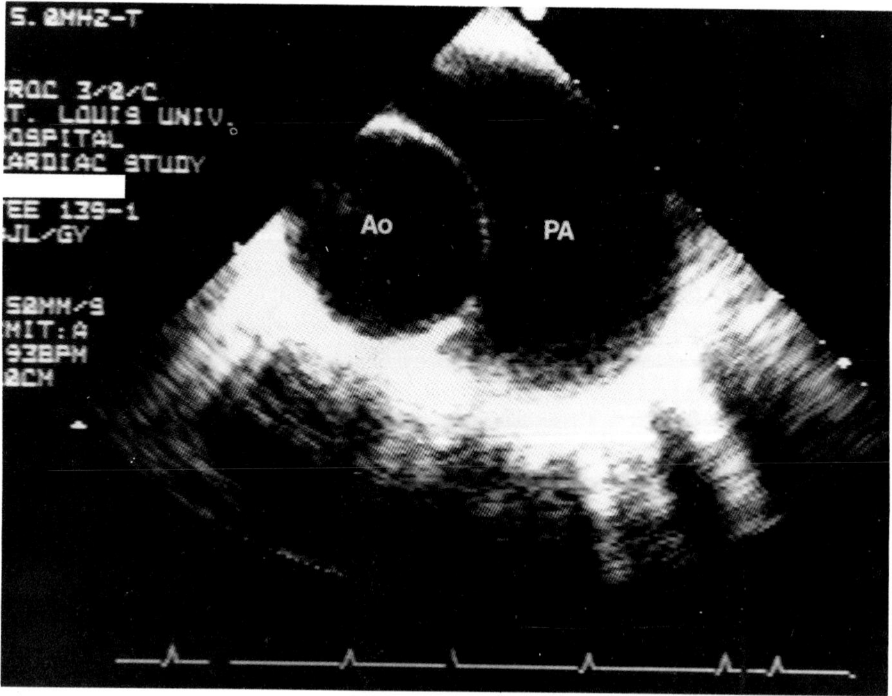

FIGURE 3-8. Main pulmonary artery (PA) near the bifurcation top as seen in basal short axis view with probe at approximately 25 cm from incisors.

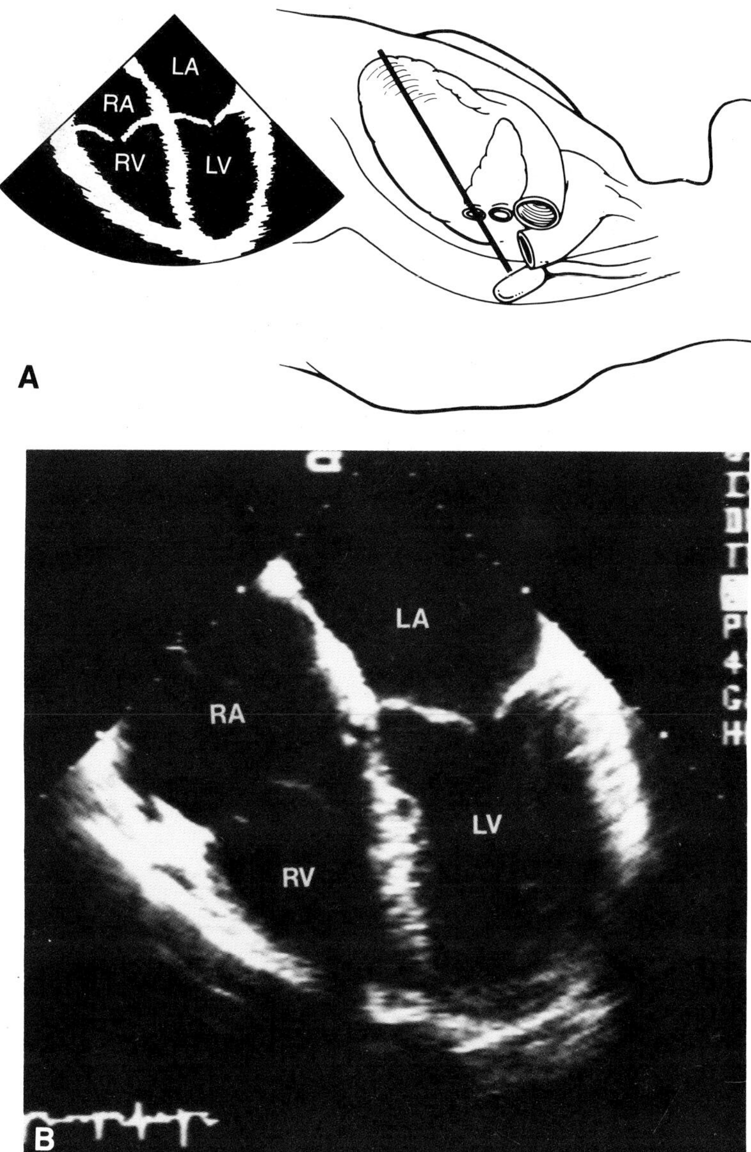

FIGURE 3-9. A. Illustration of transducer position and schematic. B. Actual image of the transesophageal four-chamber view. Note the retroflexed position of the transducer in the lower esophagus.

will allow visualization of the left ventricular outflow tract and aortic valve. Advancing and rotating the probe will allow visualization of the coronary sinus. Marked retroflexion is often needed to scan the cardiac apex in the far field.

Transgastric Short Axis View

When the probe is advanced into the stomach (40 to 45 cm), a cross-sectional image of the heart is obtained with the posterior left ventricular wall in the near field and the anterior wall in the far field (Fig. 3-10). Both left and right ventricles can now be scanned from the papillary muscle through the base of the heart as the probe is slowly withdrawn.

Thoracic Aorta

By rotating the transducer 180 degrees, one can examine the thoracic aorta (Fig. 3-11). The descending aorta is usually first appreciated in

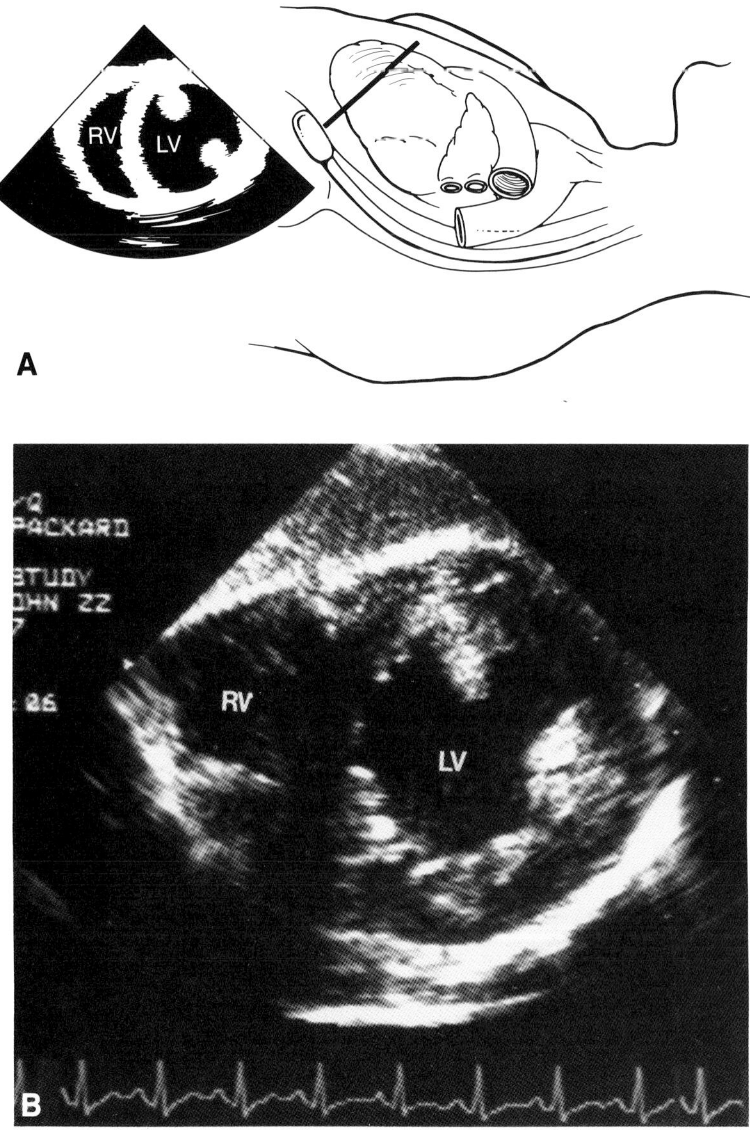

FIGURE 3-10. A. Illustration of transducer position for the gastric short axis view. B. Actual tracing demonstrating cross-sectional view of the left ventricle at the papillary muscle level. Right ventricular cavity is seen on the left side of the screen.

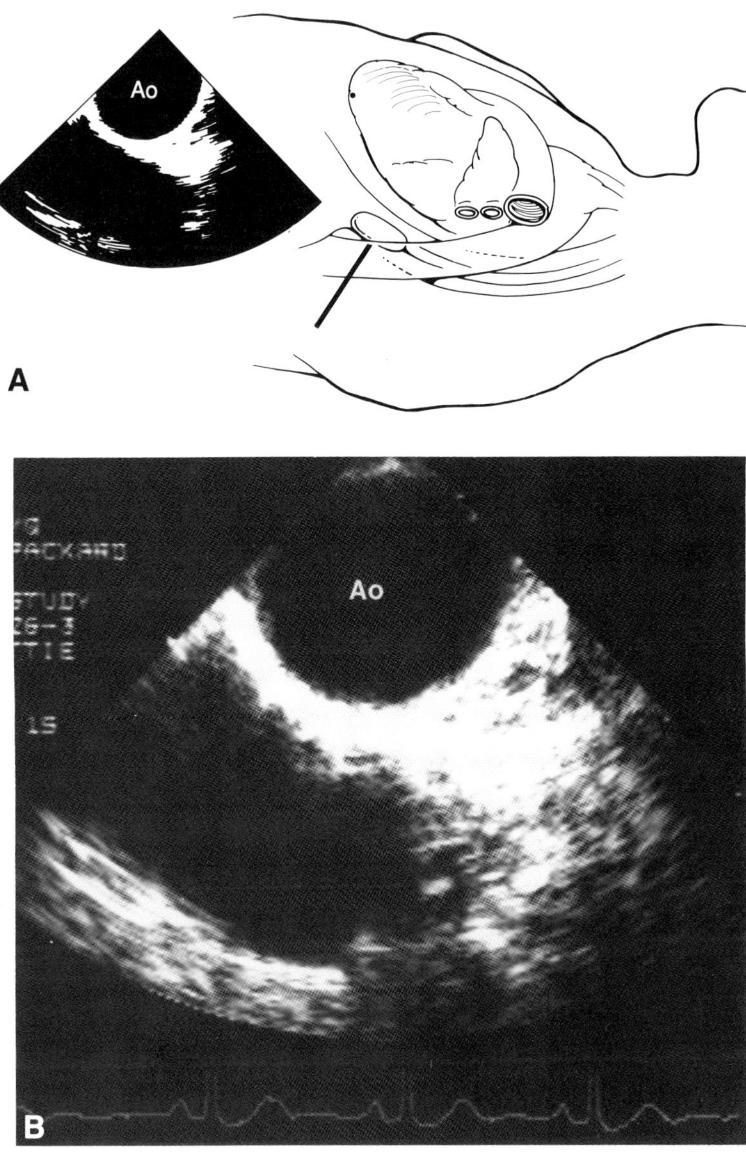

A

B

FIGURE 3-11. A. Illustration of transducer location and schematic transverse aortic image. B. Actual image obtained of the descending thoracic aorta.

the short axis view at a depth of approximately 40 cm from the incisors. The probe can then be slowly withdrawn as the descending aorta is scanned proximally. The probe is usually withdrawn to the level of the aortic arch, which can be well seen until the trachea or bronchus is interposed.

Standard Views: Biplane

Endoscopes have recently been introduced with two sets of transducers mounted on the tip with elements oriented perpendicular to each other. This has allowed imaging in the longitudinal planes, which may be of value in some patients. Imaging in the longitudinal plane is often best performed by rotating the probe in a clockwise or counterclockwise direction at several levels of the esophagus and stomach.

Gastric Views

With the probe in the stomach, the longitudinal plane will often allow long-axis visualization of a left ventricle, with the apex to the left of the screen and the mitral valve and left atrium to the right (Fig. 3-12). This view typically provides excellent definition of the inferior and anterior left ventricular free walls. By advancing the probe and then flexing the tip of the transducer, the true apex can frequently be visualized. Slight clockwise rotation of the probe in the longitudinal view will allow examination of the long axis of the right ventricle. This view provides excellent visualization of the right ventricular inflow, tricuspid subvalvular apparatus, and right ventricular apex. Rotation of the probe 180 degrees will then bring in the descending aorta. The longitudinal views of the descending thoracic aorta are helpful in rapidly assessing the presence of aortic pathology.

Esophageal Views

Longitudinal plane transesophageal examination consists of four basic orientations, with different views from each orientation (Fig. 3-13). With clockwise (moving from left side at the right-sided structures) rotation of the probe tip, these longitudinal views include (part A) left atrium and left ventricle, (part B) aorta right ventricular inflow and outflow, (part C) ascending aorta, and (part D) right atrium and vena cava. In the upper esophagus, on the left side, one can acquire views of the left atrium, mitral valve, and left ventricle. These views will demonstrate the left upper pulmonary vein, left atrium appendage, mitral valve, and left ventricle. This long-axis, two-chamber view of the left atrium and left ventricle is helpful in defining mitral valve pathology, assessing mitral regurgitation, and examining left ventricular wall motion. Slight clockwise rotation will bring the pulmonic valve, right ventricular outflow tract, and main pulmonary artery into view, depending on the level of the probe. Further clockwise rotation will reveal the ascending aorta. With flexion and withdrawal of the probe, the entire ascending aorta up to the aortic arch can often be visualized in a long-axis projection. In the lower esophagus, slight probe manip-

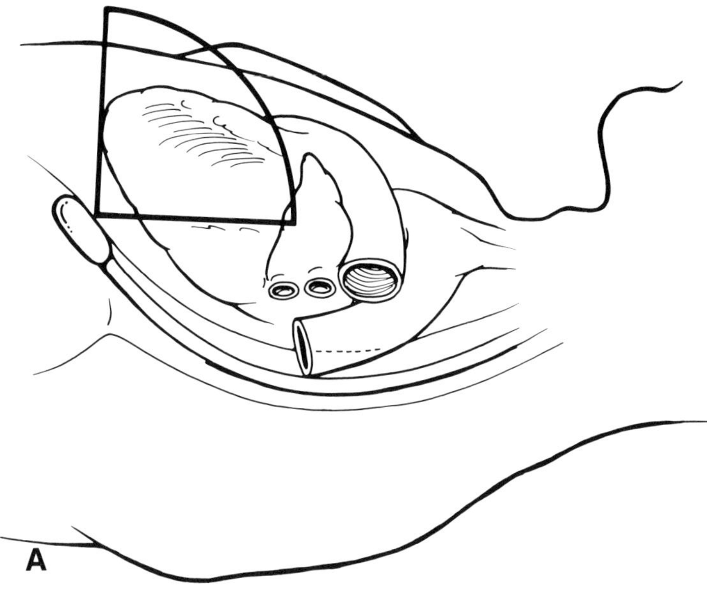

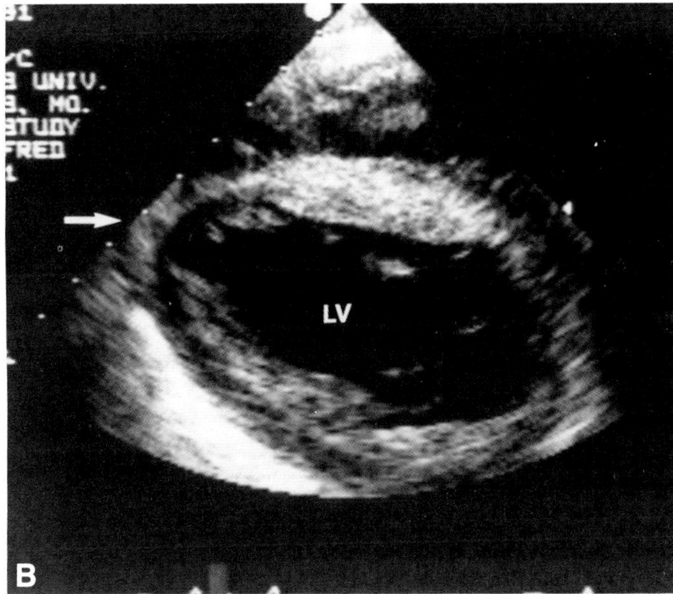

FIGURE 3-12. A. Schematic illustration of transducer location for longitudinal scan of the left ventricle with the probe in the stomach. B. This plane provides a long axis view of the left ventricle, with the posterior wall at the top of the screen and the anterior wall at the bottom of the screen. Note that this allows visualization of the cardiac apex (*arrow*).

ulation will reveal a short axis of the aortic valve, with both right ventricular inflow and outflow seen. Still further clockwise rotation of the probe tip in the upper esophagus will allow visualization of the right atrium, with its attachments to both the superior and the inferior vena cava.

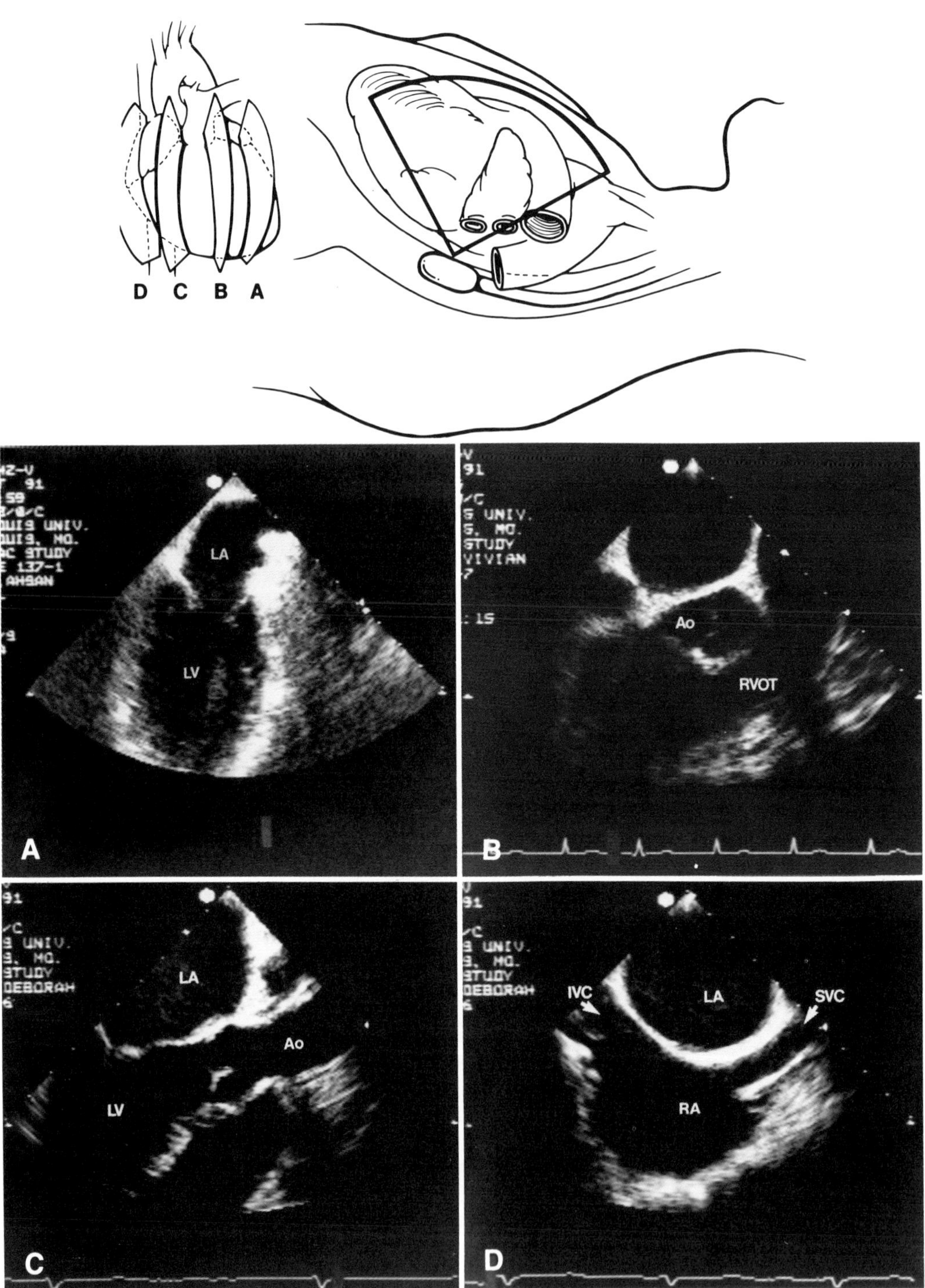

FIGURE 3-13. Top. Schematic illustration demonstrating scanning from the esophagus in a longitudinal plane in which four basic views can be obtained: A. A two-chamber view of the left atrium (LA) and left ventricle (LV), with the inferior posterior wall on the left side of the screen. B. A short axis view of the aorta (Ao), with the right ventricular inflow and outflow tract (RVOT) in the far field from left to right. C. First 3 to 5 cm of the ascending aorta (Ao) seen in the longitudinal plane. D. The right atrium with its connections both to the superior (SVC) and to the inferior (IVC) vena cava.

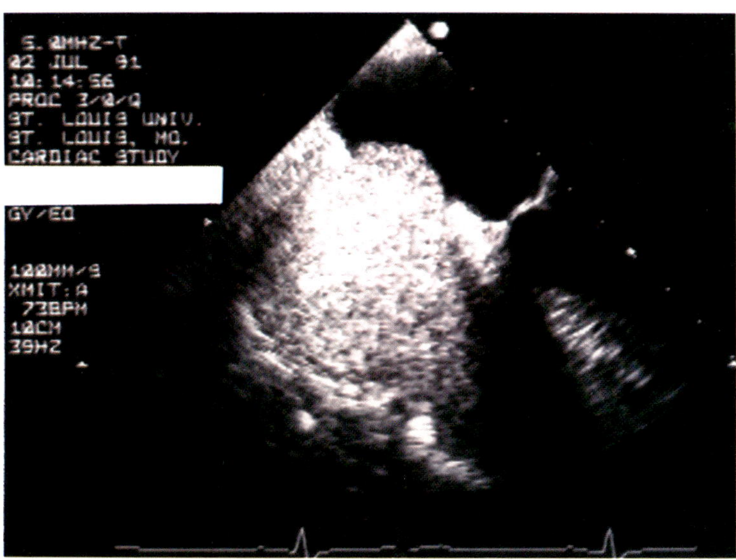

FIGURE 3-14. Opacification of the right atrium by agitated saline echo contrast material.

Contrast Enhancement

To assess for intracardiac shunting, 10 ml of agitated saline are injected rapidly through a peripheral vein. This is a routine part of the TEE examination in many laboratories (Fig. 3-14). The appearance of bubbles in the left-sided chambers within 3 to 5 beats is diagnostic for a right to left shunt. Maneuvers to increase right-sided pressures, such as cough or Valsalva maneuver, are sometimes necessary.

Risks

The risk of death associated with TEE has been reported at approximately 1 in 2500 cases. Arrhythmias, both bradycardia and tachycardia, have been reported as well. Laryngospasm, arterial hypoxemia, and inadvertent endotracheal intubation are all safety considerations. Drug reactions (intravenous sedation, antibiotics) are another potential source of morbidity. Endocarditis has been reported following TEE. Documented incidence of bacteremia is relatively low, however. Accordingly most laboratories use antibiotic prophylaxis only for prosthetic valve patients.

Bibliography

Belder, M.A., Leech, G., and Camm, A.J.: Transesophageal echocardiography in unsedated outpatients: Technique and patient tolerance. J. Am. Coll. Cardiol., *2*:375–379, 1989.

Matsuzaki, M., Toma, Y., and Kusukawa, R.: Clinical applications of transesophageal echocardiography. Circulation, *82*:709–722, 1990.

Pearson, A.C., and Pasierski, T.: Initial clinical experience with a 48 by 48 element biplane transesophageal probe. Am. Heart J., *122(2)*:559–568, 1991.

Richardson, S.G., Weintraub, A.R., Schwartz, S.L., et al.: Biplane transesophageal echocardiography utilizing transverse and sagittal imaging planes. Echocardiography, *8(3)*:293, 1991.

Seward, J.B., Khandheria, I.K., Oh, J.K., et al.: Transesophageal echocardiography: Technique, anatomic correlations, implementation and clinical applications. Mayo Clin. Proc., *63*:649–680, 1988.

Zabalgoitia, M., Gandhi, D.K., Evans, J., et al.: Transesophageal echocardiography in the awake elderly patient: Its role in the clinical decision-making process. Am. Heart J., *120*:1147–1153, 1990.

4

TEE in Critically Ill Patients

Echocardiography has long played a crucial role in the evaluation of the critically ill patient. The portability, widespread availability, and instantaneous diagnostic capability of ultrasound equipment make it ideal for the assessment of critically ill patients. The utility of surface cross-sectional Doppler echocardiography has been demonstrated in the assessment of complications of myocardial infarction, pericardial effusion, and cardiac tamponade; in the detection of aortic dissection; in the evaluation of cardiogenic embolic sources; and in noninvasive determinations of the presence and severity of valvular pathologic conditions. Because the equipment used for echocardiography is portable, echocardiographic studies can be performed at bedside within minutes of a change in clinical status. Studies are read on-line, and the results are immediately available without any further computer processing. Because ultrasound units are relatively inexpensive and harmless, serial studies can be performed to assess response to therapy. The major limitation to echocardiography has been the need for a good acoustic window. In critically ill patients, appropriate imaging is frequently limited because of wounds or tubing that block transducer access. In addition, lack of patient cooperation and the inability to move patients into the left lateral decubitus position contributes to a high prevalence of technically inadequate studies.

With TEE, the advantages of echocardiography in the evaluation of critically ill patients are retained. Within 15 minutes of a request, the study can be initiated at bedside. Furthermore the images are always excellent because of the location of the ultrasound probe in the esophagus, contiguous to the left atrium, which obviates the acoustic interference from structures of the chest wall. The availability of TEE for examination of patients in the intensive care unit has greatly enhanced our ability to manage critically ill patients.

Certain methodologic differences between the performance of TEE in the ambulatory, stable patient and the critically ill, intensive care

TABLE 4-1. TEE in the Critically Ill Patient

Shorter acting sedative/narcotic
Paralyzing agents when appropriate
Very liberal sedation/anesthesia if dissection is suspected
Goal-directed examination
Ventilated patients
Paralytic ileus

unit patient must be kept in mind (Table 4-1). First, the critically ill patient may require different sedative/anesthetic combinations. Shorter acting narcotic agents are preferred for analgesia (morphine versus meperidine [Demerol]) and shorter acting benzodiazepine agents (midazolam versus diazepam) for sedation when blood pressure respirations or mental states are tenuous. In the patient with borderline respiratory status and significant tachypnea, carbon dioxide retention, or hypoxemia, even a small amount of sedative may be enough to cause respiratory failure. Consequently in these patients we encourage delay of TEE until either the patient's respiratory status has considerably improved or the patient is intubated and ventilation is mechanically supported. Almost all critically ill patients are best examined while being monitored by pulsed oximetry. Such continuous monitoring allows early action or termination of the procedure if desaturation occurs. Because respiratory arrest is not a concern in patients who are receiving ventilatory support, these patients can be given sedative/narcotic agents more liberally as long as blood pressure is stable. Newer neuromuscular paralyzing agents (pancuronium, vecuronium) may be necessary in the uncooperative patient who is already receiving ventilatory support. Adequate sedation should be given whenever neuromuscular paralyzing agents are administered. Intravenous vecuronium, with its shorter half-life and earlier onset of action, is particularly useful for performing TEE (Table 4-2).

Of particular concern are patients in whom aortic dissection is suspected. Any undue stress caused by the passage of the TEE probe could lead to increased catecholamine production, with a resultant increase in cardiac contractility and exacerbation of the dissection. Therefore patients with suspected aortic dissection should be given liberal

TABLE 4-2. Vecuronium (NORCURON) for ICU-TEE Anesthesia

For noncooperative ventilator patients
Nondepolarizing neuromuscular blocking agents
Competes for cholinergic receptors at motor end-plate
$\frac{1}{3}$ more potent than pancuronium (Pavulon) with shorter duration
   (20–30 min)
0.08 to 0.10 mg/kg (5–10 mg) IV bolus
Give with sedative

amounts of sedation and analgesia. The aim should be to induce a highly sedated, almost somnolent state during which probe passage can be accomplished without agitation.

The second major difference between standard TEE examinations and the TEE examination in critically ill patients is the need for goal-directed examinations in the latter. In patients with suspected aortic dissection, for example, the examination should be immediately directed toward the proximal aorta to rule out a type I dissection, followed quickly by a scan of the descending aorta to rule out type III dissection. This approach allows the diagnosis to be ruled in or out within 30 to 60 seconds, and the rest of the examination can be done more thoroughly and meticulously. If a complication then develops or the patient is unable to tolerate the probe, the diagnosis is secure.

The third unique aspect of TEE in the intensive care unit is the examination of the ventilated patient. As previously discussed, sedative/analgesic agents may need to be modified. In addition, the presence of a protected airway allows examinations to be performed in the supine position. We usually perform these examinations on the right side of the bed with the ultrasound machine on the left, thus allowing easy manipulation of the probe and visualization of the ultrasound screen. Passage of the probe is accomplished using manual guidance in the usual fashion. Occasionally esophageal intubation cannot be accomplished blindly, and direct laryngoscopic visualization of the esophagus is employed.

Finally, critically ill patients frequently develop paralytic ileus of the intestines. Thus despite the absence of food or nasogastric feedings, a large amount of gastric contents may be present. Although most ventilator patients will have nasogastric tubes in place, providing low-pressure intermittent suction to ensure empty stomachs, this is not necessarily the case in other critically ill patients. Abdominal examination should be performed before esophageal intubation, and if there is evidence for paralytic ileus, a nasogastric tube should be inserted to empty the stomach.

With these special considerations in mind, the TEE examination can be performed safely and effectively in 99% of critically ill patients.

Indications

We have reported on our early experience with TEE in critically ill patients, and our subsequent experience with over 200 examinations is similar to this early report. The bulk of our examinations are performed in a coronary care unit setting (49%), with the remainder distributed between postoperative cardiothoracic intensive care units (21%), the general medical intensive care unit (19%), and the general surgery/trauma units (11%). The distribution of indications for imaging is shown in Figure 4-1.

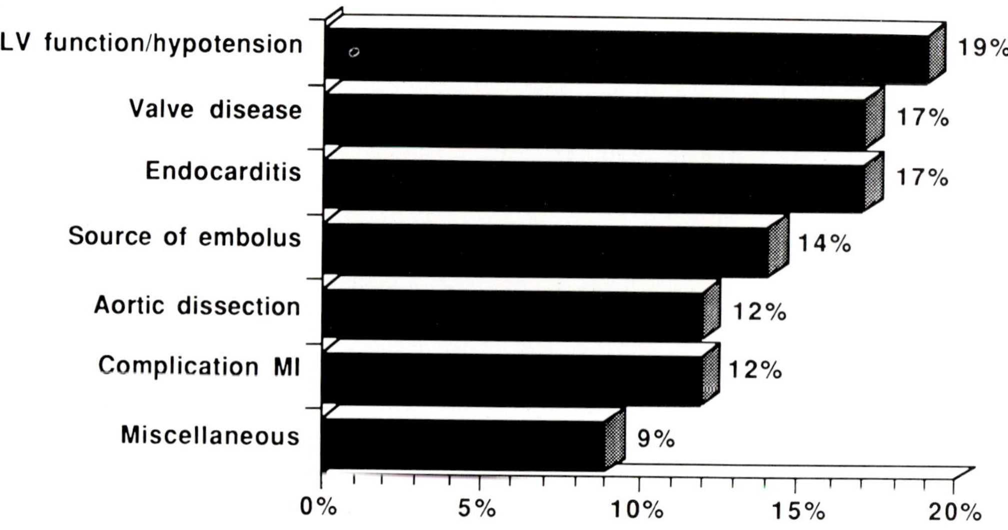

FIGURE 4-1. Indications for TEE imaging in the intensive care unit in an active laboratory.

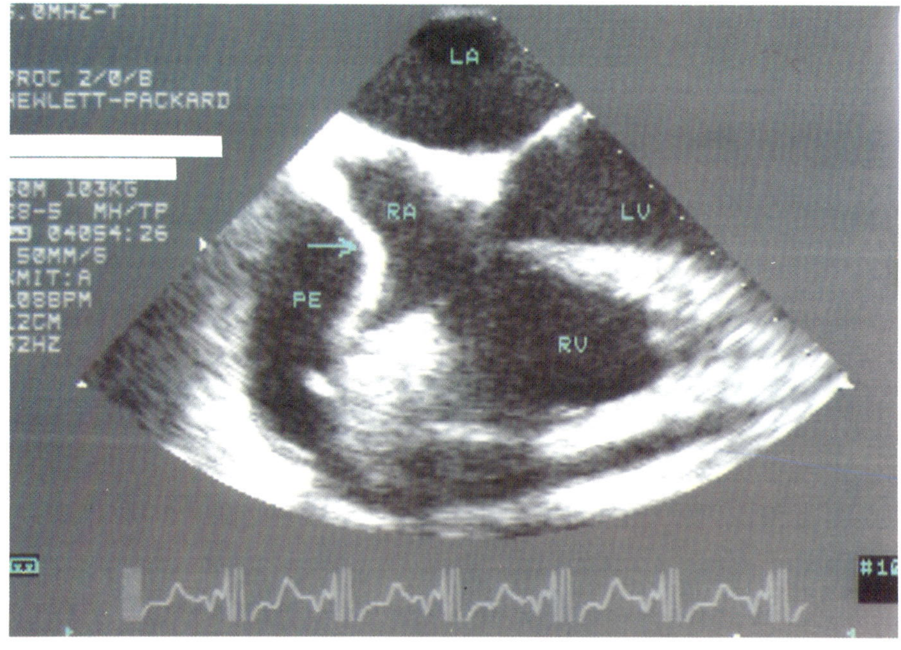

FIGURE 4-2. Right atrial collapse consistent with tamponade physiology (*arrow*) in a patient with a moderate size pericardial effusion (PE) and hypotension.

Left Ventricular Function/Hypotension

The most common indication for TEE in the intensive care unit in our experience has been for assessment of left ventricular function. In the critically ill patient with unexplained hypotension in whom surface echo is technically inadequate, TEE provides critical bedside information that can determine the contribution of (1) cardiac tamponade (Fig. 4-2), (2) left ventricular dysfunction (Fig. 4-3), (3) hypovolemia, or (4) valvular disease to hemodynamic compromise. In patients with unexplained hypoxemia, TEE is useful for excluding occult right to left shunts caused by patent foramen ovale or atrial septal defect. In many patients, information on the cardiac contribution to hypotension or pulmonary edema can be gained from echocardiography. When echocardiographic examination is limited, TEE can provide critical information on right and left ventricular volumes, systolic function, and valvular function.

Valve Disease

Another common indication for imaging in the intensive care unit is for assessment of native or prosthetic valve disease. Auscultation and clinical examination can be limited in the intensive care unit owing

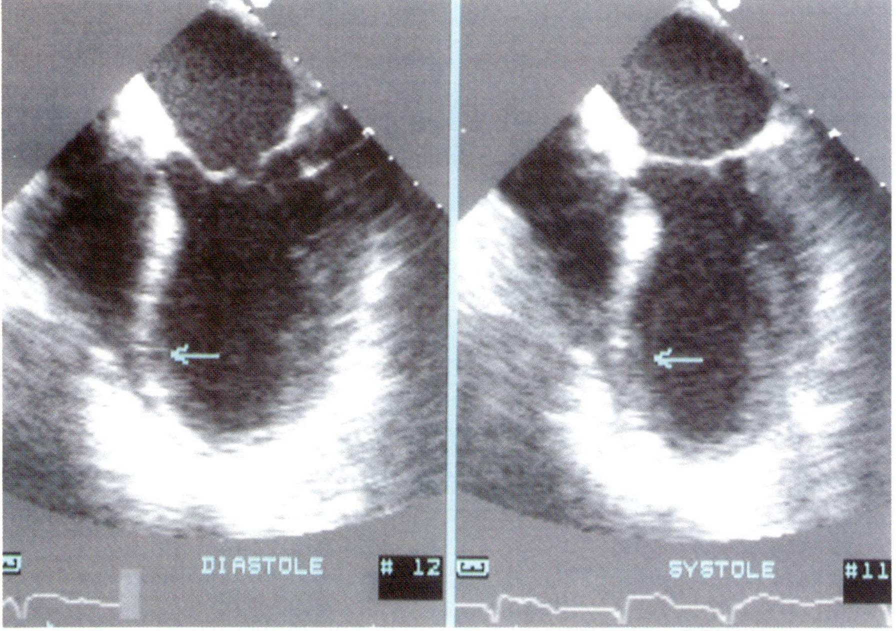

FiGURE 4-3. Four-chamber view in diastole (left panel) and systole (right panel), indicating large area of septal and apical akinesis (*arrow*). Imaging was done to assess cardiac function in a patient with unexplained hypotension and hypoxemia.

to multiple factors. TEE is extremely helpful in sorting out the contribution of valvular dysfunction to either hypotension or hypoxemia.

Aortic Pathology

The majority of examinations for aortic pathology have been performed in the coronary care unit in patients with chest pain and suspected aortic dissection. Not uncommonly, patients present with chest pain and nonspecific electrocardiographic changes. Under these circumstances, TEE can rapidly differentiate between aortic dissection and unstable angina or myocardial infarction. If aortic dissection can be confidently and rapidly ruled out at the bedside, intravenous heparin or thrombolytic therapy can be given for presumed ischemic coronary disease. Identification of new or changing wall motion abnormalities aids further in the diagnosis of ischemic syndromes. Not uncommonly, TEE will discover other noncardiac causes of chest pain and aid in their definition (Fig. 4-4).

TEE may also prove useful in the assessment of patients who have suffered severe blunt chest trauma. A large percentage of these patients are sent for aortic angiography to rule out aortic rupture. TEE can quickly assess for this entity at the bedside.

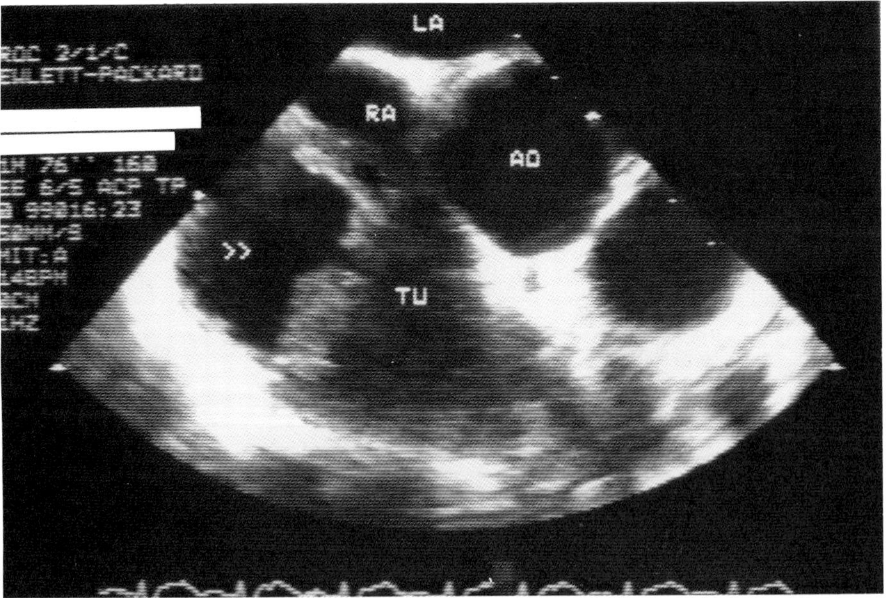

FIGURE 4-4. Large tumor (TU) with areas of liquefaction (*arrowheads*) compressing the right atrium in a patient with chest pain and nonspecific ECG changes.

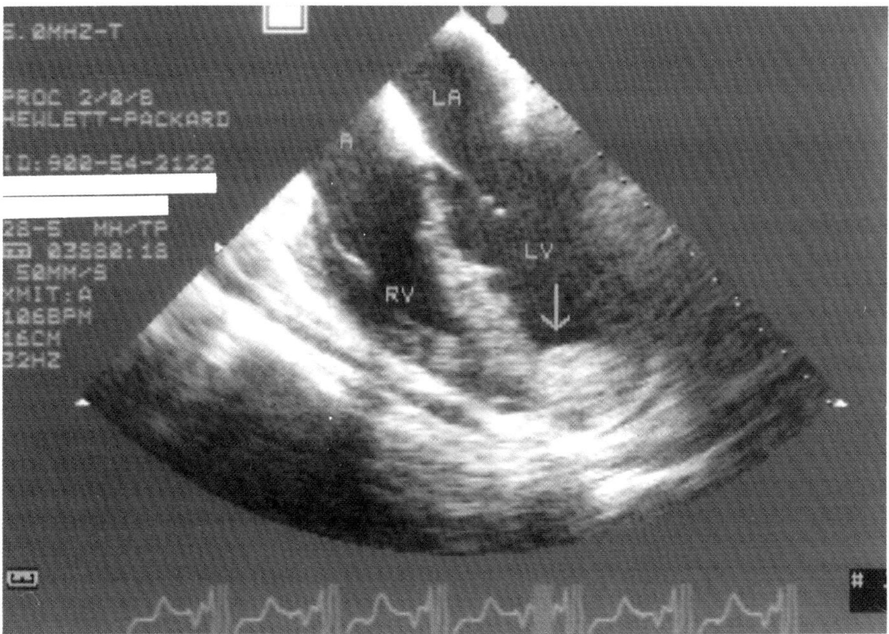

Figure 4-5. Large apical thrombus (*arrow*) identified solely by TEE.

Cardiac Source of Embolus

Another common indication for TEE in our experience in critically ill patients is to rule out a cardiac source of embolus. We have identified atrial thrombus in approximately 25% of such patients that has not been evident from surface echocardiography. In addition, TEE can identify shunting across a patent foramen ovale or atrial septal defect that may be responsible for paradoxical embolus, atrial septal aneurysms, and apical thrombus (Fig. 4-5).

We have found TEE particularly useful in patients with pulmonary embolus. In these patients, TEE can exclude right atrial thrombus and actually identify embolus in the pulmonary artery.

Complications of Myocardial Infarction

Several investigators have reported on the utility of TEE in the patient with myocardial infarction. TEE has proved accurate in detecting papillary muscle rupture (Fig. 4-6) and can clearly identify both the detached head of the papillary muscle flailing into the left atrium and the severe mitral regurgitation associated with it. In many cases when coronary anatomy is already known, we have been able to take the patient directly to the operating room following TEE. In addition, reports indicate TEE may be more accurate than surface echocardiogra-

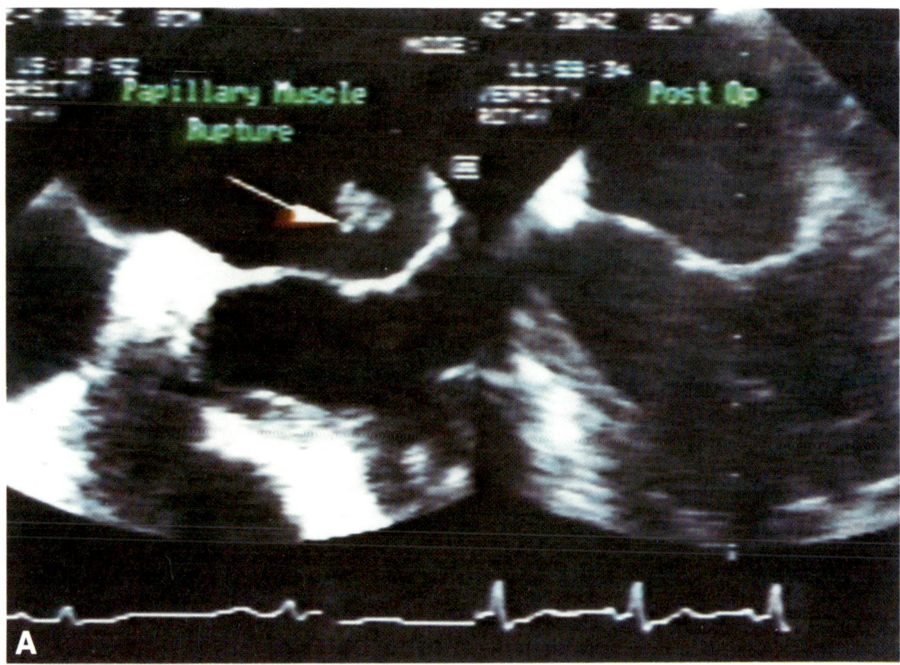

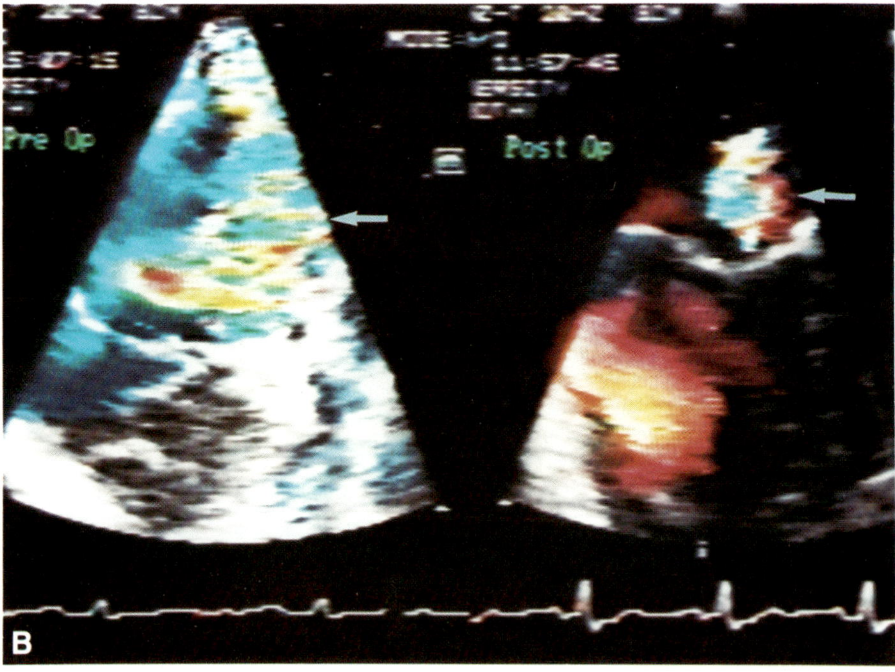

FIGURE 4-6. A. (Left) Rupture of the papillary muscle head (*arrow*) in a patient with new murmur and pulmonary edema following acute inferior myocardial infarction (MI), and (right) patient after mitral valve repair. B. (Left) Color flow imaging demonstrating severe mitral regurgitation (*arrow*) in a patient with a papillary muscle head rupture, and (right) following mitral valve repair, only a small color flow jet (*arrow*) consistent with mild mitral regurgitation is noted.

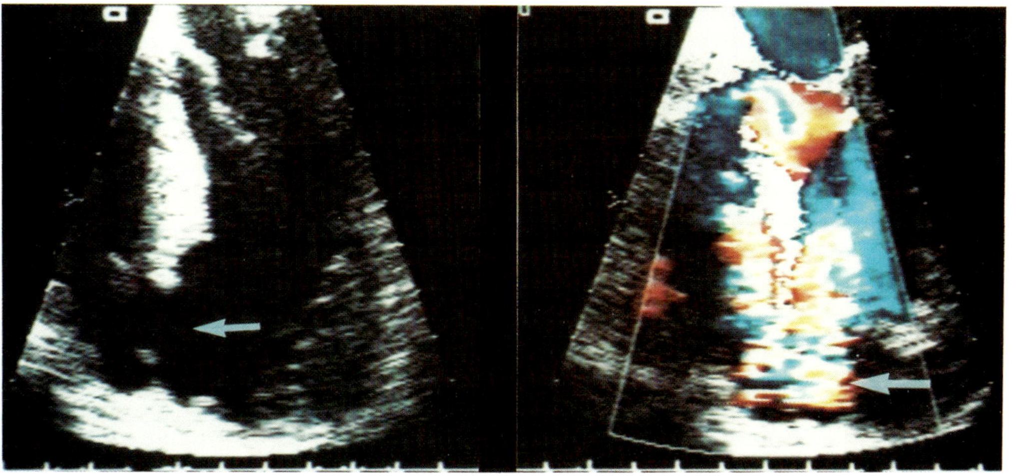

FIGURE 4-7. TEE image (left) and color flow (right) demonstrating a large anteroapical ventricular septal defect (*arrow*) 3 days post–myocardial infarction.

phy for localizing and characterizing other mechanical complications of myocardial infarction, including ventricular septal defect (Fig. 4-7), aneurysm (Fig. 4-8), and pseudoaneurysm (Fig. 4-9).

We have reported on several unique diagnostic entities complicating myocardial infarction where TEE was particularly useful. One patient

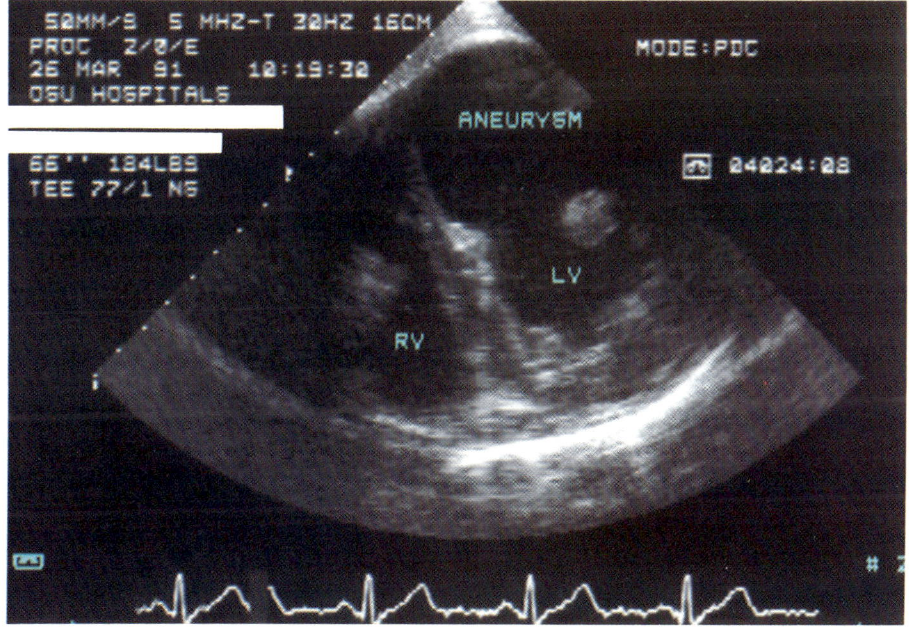

FIGURE 4-8. Large inferoposterior aneurysm identified by transgastric transesophageal imaging.

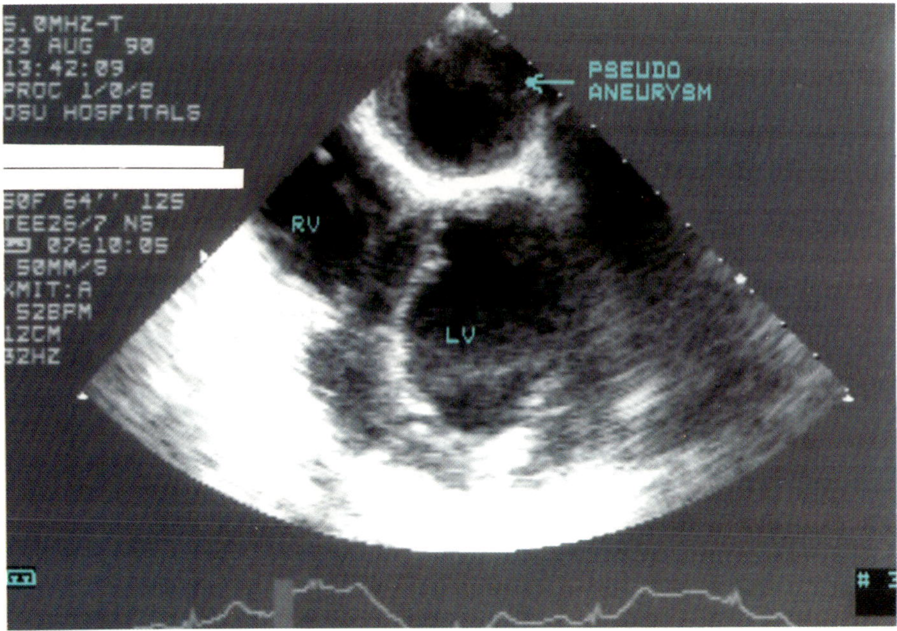

FIGURE 4-9. Transgastric short-axis view of left ventricle (LV) demonstrating pseudoaneurysm secondary to inferior myocardial infarction. Note inferior wall akinesis and thrombus partially filling the pseudoaneurysm.

developed a loud systolic murmur and large V-waves associated with arterial hypotension and pulmonary edema one day after percutaneous transluminal coronary angioplasty of a circumflex coronary artery lesion. Although the surface echocardiogram did not provide a diagnosis, TEE revealed severe mitral regurgitation and turbulence in the left ventricular outflow tract consistent with hypertrophic obstructive cardiomyopathy (Fig. 4-10). The left ventricle was severely hypertrophied and hyperdynamic. This patient died during surgery to correct the mitral regurgitation, and severe hypertrophic cardiomyopathy was confirmed at autopsy.

TEE may also be useful in the diagnosis of right atrial infarction complicating right ventricular infarction by a triad of right atrial spontaneous contrast, atrial akinesis, and lack of atrial peak on tricuspid inflow (Fig. 4-11).

Cardiothoracic Intensive Care Imaging

The postoperative cardiac surgery patient represents a unique challenge for surface echocardiography. A high proportion of such studies are technically inadequate because of postoperative changes from sternotomy or thoracotomy or because of limited window from chest tubes, dressings, and sutures. Most particularly, however, in these patients,

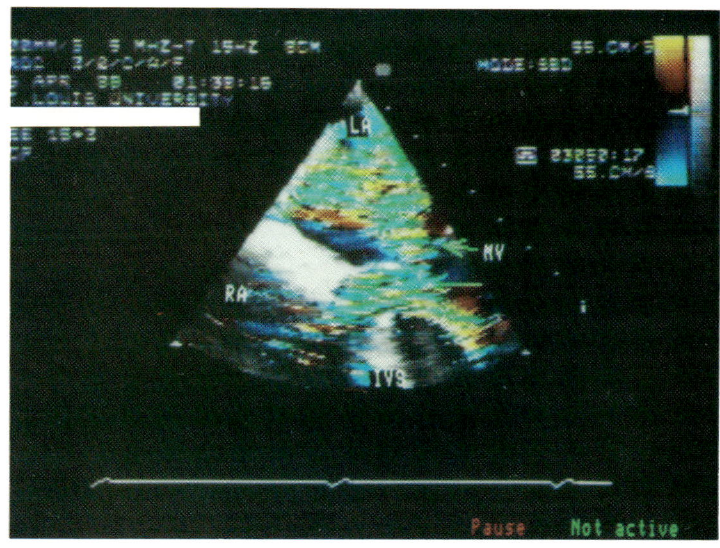

FIGURE 4-10. Four-chamber imaging from upper esophagus indicating severe mitral regurgitation and heavy turbulence in the left ventricular outflow tract as a result of systolic anterior motion of the mitral valve.

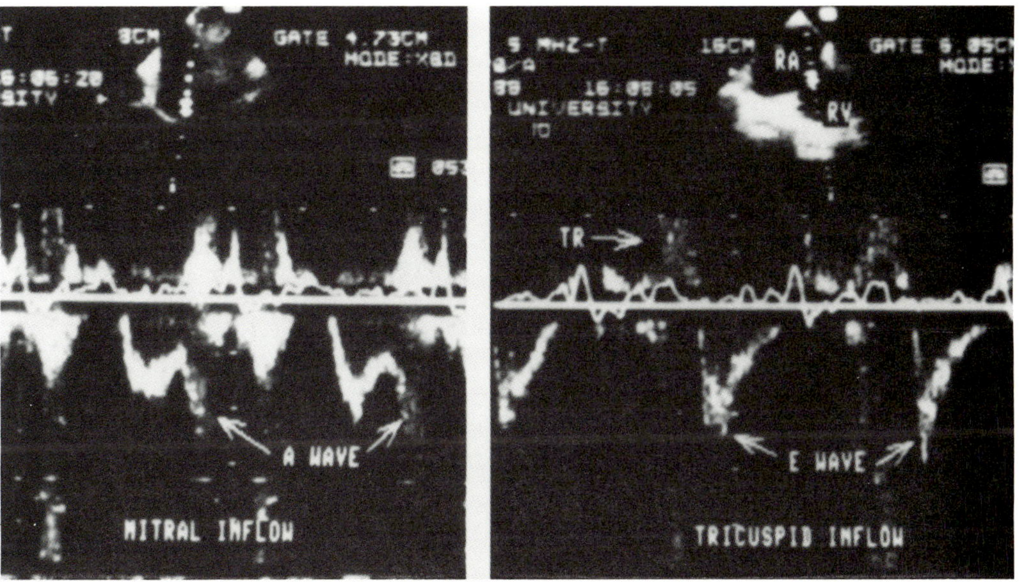

FIGURE 4-11. Pulsed Doppler of mitral inflow on the left in patient in cardiogenic shock demonstrating normal A-waves. Near-simultaneous Doppler of tricuspid inflow demonstrating absent A-waves as a result of right atrial infarction on the right.

quick, noninvasive diagnosis of native or prosthetic valve dysfunction, left ventricular dysfunction, or cardiac tamponade is most essential. TEE fulfills this role nicely (Fig. 4-12).

In particular, experience indicates the utility of detecting right atrial compression caused by hematoma in these patients. In suspected pulmonary embolus, TEE can aid in identification of right atrial thrombus (Fig. 4-13).

Other Indications

TEE can be useful in the diagnosis of infective endocarditis in the intensive care unit. In particular, critically ill patients with prosthetic valves are better assessed by TEE than by surface echocardiography. In patients following valve replacement procedures, TEE provides unique information on valve function, abscess formation, and fistula formation.

Safety

TEE examinations in the intensive care unit when done with appropriate consideration for the special inherent circumstances can be per-

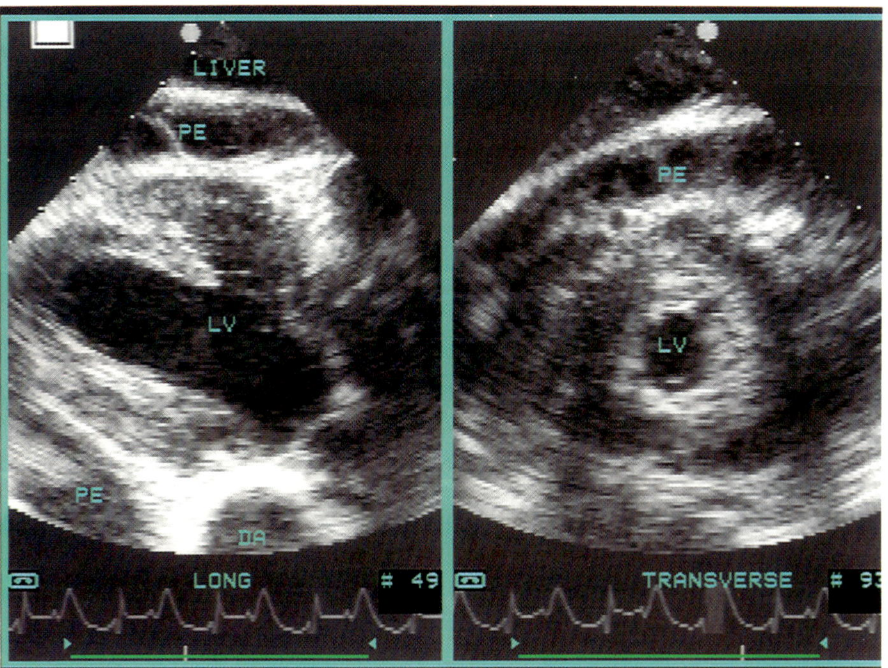

FIGURE 4-12. Transgastric imaging in longitudinal plane (left) and transverse plane (right) demonstrating large pericardial hematoma (PE) after open-heart surgery causing cardiac compression. (DA = descending aorta.)

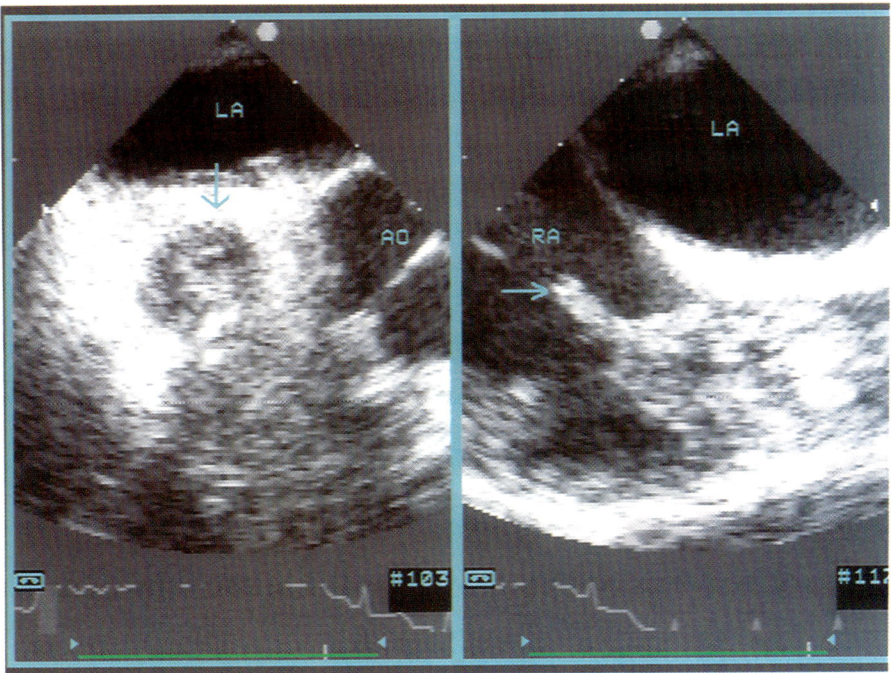

FIGURE 4-13. Transverse plane imaging at basal short axis level in a patient with multiple pulmonary emboli (left). The superior vena cava (*arrow*) is filled with thrombus. (Right) The longitudinal plane demonstrates length of the thrombus as it protrudes (*arrow*) into the body of the right atrium (RA). (AO = Aorta.)

formed with remarkably few complications. There have been no reported cases of aspiration pneumonia or esophageal perforation and no mortalities to date. In our reported series of 62 examinations, three complications occurred. One patient with a seizure disorder and inadequate phenytoin levels developed a grand mal seizure during the examination, which resolved after treatment without sequelae. One patient vomited gastric contents without lung aspiration.

Conclusions

TEE can be performed safely in critically ill patients. The major indications in the intensive care unit for performing TEE are (1) evaluating aortic pathologic conditions, (2) ruling out cardiac source of embolus, (3) evaluating the patient with myocardial infarction, and (4) diagnosing infective endocarditis and its complications.

Bibliography

Abrams, D.S., Starling, M.R., Crawford, M.H., and O'Rourke, R.A.: Value of noninvasive techniques for predicting early complications in patients with clinical class II acute myocardial infarction. J. Am. Coll. Cardiol., 2:818–825, 1983.

Blondheim, D.S., Jacobs, L.E., Kotler, M.N., et al.: Anterolateral myocardial rupture following mitral valve replacement: Transesophageal echo documentation of ischemic etiology. Am. Heart J. 119(3):681–683, 1990.

Callahan, J.A., Seward, J.B., Nishimura, R.A., et al.: Two-dimensional echocardiographically guided pericardiocentesis: Experience in 117 consecutive patients. Am. J. Cardiol., 55:476–479, 1985.

DePace, N.L., Soulen, R.L., Kotler, M.N., and Mintz, G.S.: Two dimensional echocardiography detection of intraatrial masses. Am. J. Cardiol., 48:954–960, 1981.

Feigenbaum, H.: Acquried valvular heart disease. *In* Echocardiography. Edited by H. Felgenbaum. 4th ed. Philadelphia, Lea & Febiger, 1986, pp 249–364.

Hilton, T.C.: Acute mitral regurgitation with cardiogenic shock in a patient with hypertrophic cardiomyopathy: A critical management dilemma. Am. Heart J., 119(5):1205–1207, 1990.

Hilton, T.C., Pearson, A.C., Serota, H., et al.: Right atrial infarction and cardiogenic shock complicating acute myocardial infarction: Diagnosis by transesophageal echocardiography. Am. Heart J., 120(2):427–430, 1990.

Issacsohn, J.L., Earle, M.G., Kemper, A.J., and Parisi, A.F.: Postmyocardial infarction pain and infarct extension in the coronary care unit. Role of two-dimensional echocardiography. J. Am. Coll. Cardiol., 11:246–251, 1988.

Khandheria, B.K., Tajik, A.J., Taylor, C.L., et al.: Aortic dissection: Review of value and limitations of two-dimensional echocardiography in a six-year experience. J. Am. Soc. Echo., 2:17–24, 1989.

Kochar, G.S., Jacobs, L.E., and Kotler, M.N.: Right atrial compression in postoperative cardiac patients: Detection by transesophageal echocardiography. J. Am. Coll. Cardiol., 16(2):511–516, 1990.

Mathew, T., and Nanda, N.C.: Two-dimensional and Doppler echocardiography evaluation of aortic aneurysm and dissection. Am. J. Cardiol., 54:379–385, 1984.

Nixdorf, U., Erbel, R., Drexler, K., and Meyer, J.: Detection of thromboembolus of the right pulmonary artery by transesophageal two-dimensional echocardiography. Am. J. Cardiol., 61:488–489, 1988.

Oh, J.K., Seward, J.B., and Khandheria, B.K.: Transesophageal echocardiography in the intensive care unit (abstract). Circulation, 78(suppl II):II–298, 1988.

Parisi, A.F., Moynihan, P.E., Folland, E.D., et al.: Echocardiography in acute and remote myocardial infarction. Am. J. Cardiol., 46:1205–1214, 1980.

Pearson, A.C., Castello, R., Labovitz, A.J., et al.: Safety and utility of transesophageal echocardiography in the critically ill patient. Am. Heart J., 119:1083–1089, 1990.

Stoddard, M.F., Keedy, D.L., and Kupersmith, J.: Transesophageal echocardiographic diagnosis of papillary muscle rupture complicating acute myocardial infarction. Am. Heart J., 120(3):690–692, 1990.

Wittlich, N., Erbel, R., Todt, M., et al.: Detection of pulmonary artery thrombi by transesophageal echocardiography in patients with suspected pulmonary embolism (abstract). J. Am. Coll. Cardiol., 13:224A, 1989.

5

Intraoperative TEE

Epicardial echocardiography has been used in the intraoperative management of cardiac surgical patients for almost a decade. Widespread acceptance of the technique, however, has been limited for a variety of reasons: (1) Until the advent of color flow Doppler, there was no reasonably accurate, widely applicable ultrasound method for assessment of valvular insufficiency. (2) Application of *epicardial* transducers requires invasion of the surgical field and proficiency of a surgeon in imaging. Thus the development of TEE probes with color flow Doppler capabilities represented a major advance in the field. The explosion of interest in and performance of intraoperative TEE is an obvious testimonial to this advance.

In adults, there are two major areas where TEE has been applied intraoperatively: (1) in the intraoperative cardiac monitoring of the noncardiac surgical patient and (2) in the postoperative assessment of valve repair. In children with congenital heart disease, TEE is being used more widely as smaller and smaller probes are developed.

Intraoperative Techniques

The technique of probe insertion in the anesthetized patient varies only slightly from that of the ambulatory patient. The probe is advanced manually and usually without direct visualization into the posterior pharynx. Midline position is ensured by digital examination. Generally in the anesthetized patient, gentle pressure allows the probe tip to pass into the esophagus without difficulty. Positioning in the esophagus can be confirmed by good visualization of the left atrium and aortic valve. If difficulty is encountered, we use direct laryngoscopic visualization to advance the probe tip into proper position.

A full examination is usually performed to exclude major structural cardiac abnormalities. For monitoring during the operation, the probe is advanced into the stomach and transgastric short-axis view at the papillary muscle level obtained. This view allows visualization of myocardial segments perfused by the three major coronary arteries and thus is the optimal single view for detection of ischemia. In addition, the short-axis view is more sensitive than long-axis dimensions to alterations in left ventricular filling caused by hypovolemia.

Monitoring Left Ventricular Function

Cardiac function and ischemia during noncardiac surgery have traditionally been monitored by measuring arterial and pulmonary capillary wedge pressures along with electrocardiography. Recent studies indicate that TEE monitoring of cardiac function may be a superior method for on-line assessment of left ventricular global and regional systolic function, filling, and ischemia.

By monitoring the cross-sectional area in the short-axis view, a measure of left ventricular filling that may be superior to pulmonary capillary wedge pressure is obtained, and by observing the reduction in cross-sectional area, an estimate of ejection fraction is available on-

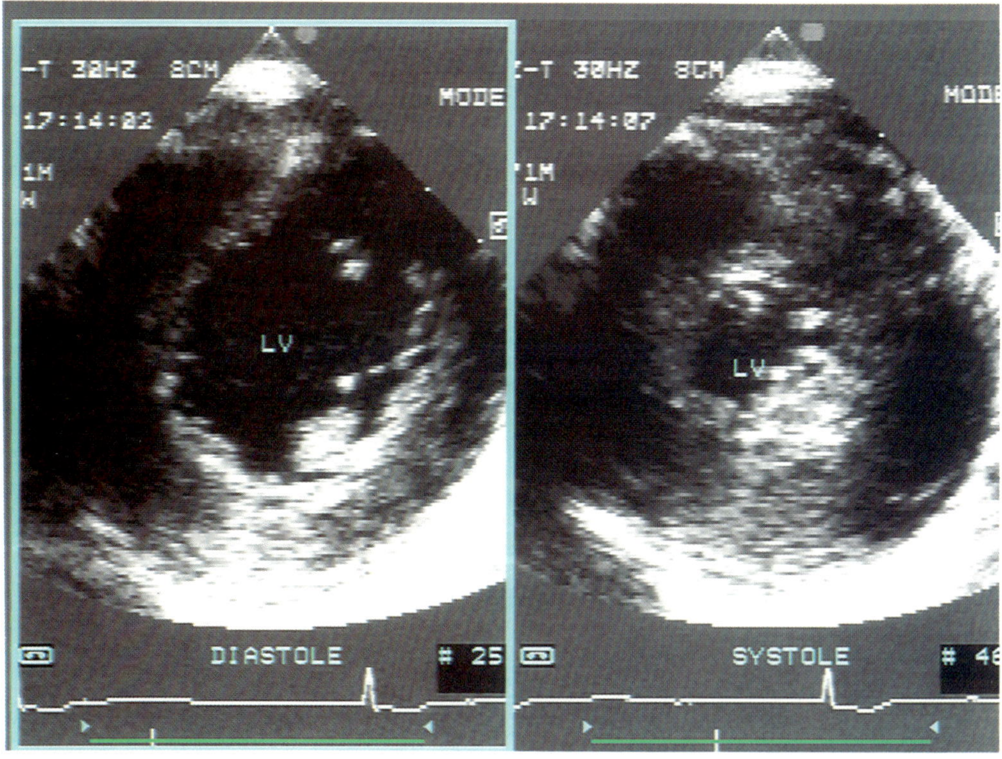

FIGURE 5-1. Transgastric recordings of small, hyperdynamic left ventricle (LV) in a hypotensive patient.

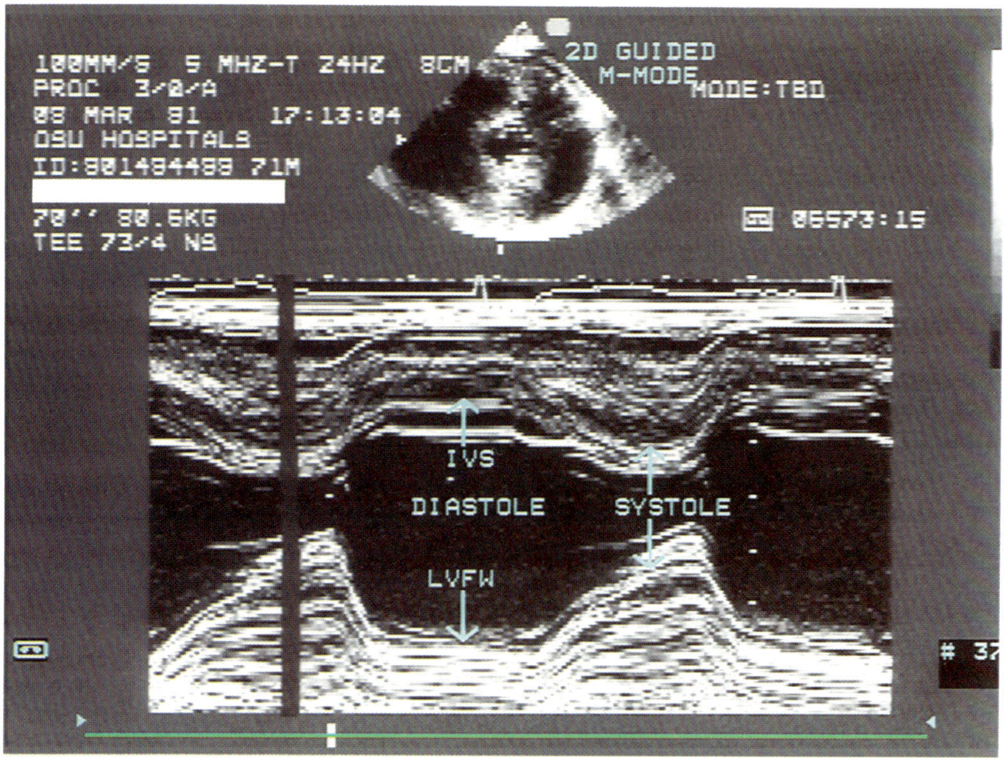

FIGURE 5-2. Transgastric intraoperative M-mode recordings from a hypotensive patient demonstrating small left ventricular cavity size at end-diastole with increased shortening during systole. (IVS = Ventricular septum; LVFW = left ventricular free wall.)

line. Echocardiographic estimates of ejection fraction obtained in this manner have been shown to correlate well with simultaneously obtained radionuclide estimates ($r = 0.96$). The availability of a digital cine-loop image of the baseline short-axis views aids greatly in the intraoperative assessment of changes in left ventricular volume and ejection performance. Intraoperative hypotension may be due to inadequate filling of the left ventricle despite normal wedge pressure readings (Figs. 5-1 and 5-2).

Numerous studies have documented that one of the earliest signs of ischemia is the cessation of regional cardiac muscle contraction. Thus intraoperative monitoring of left ventricular function should be theoretically a sensitive method for the early detection of ischemia. TEE detects ischemia as manifested by regional wall motion abnormalities three to four times as often as detected by electrocardiographic changes. In addition, persistent regional wall motion abnormalities identified by TEE are an important prognostic sign for subsequently documented cardiovascular complications (Fig. 5-3).

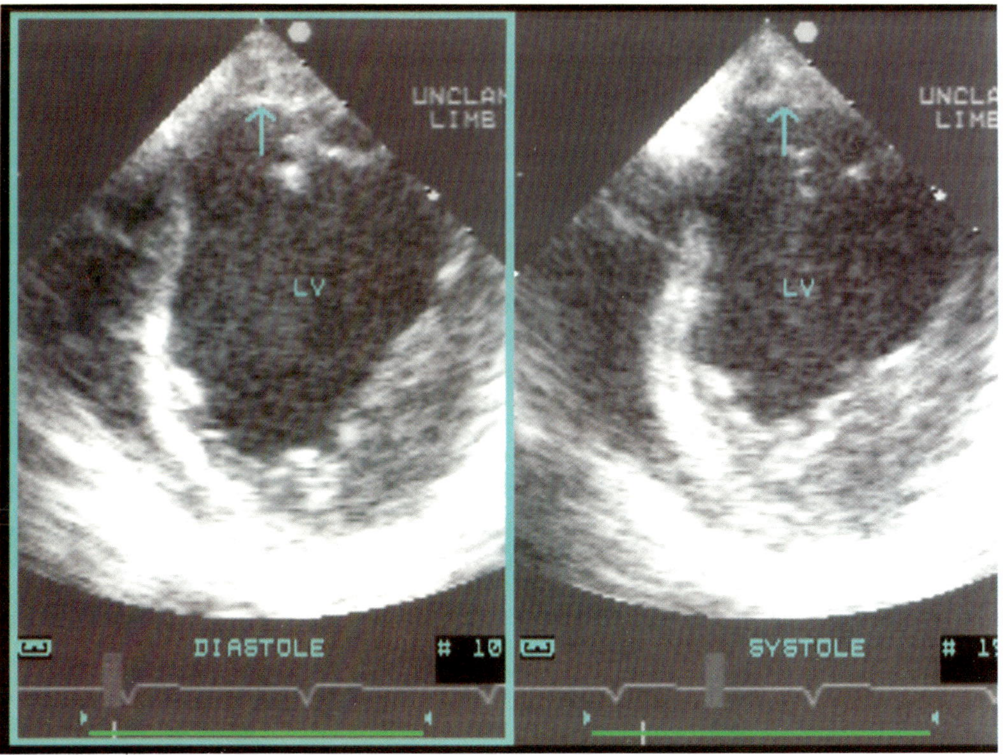

FIGURE 5-3. Intraoperative transgastric short-axis TEE recording in diastole (left) and systole (right) demonstrating inferior dyskinesis.

TEE for Mitral Valve Repair

One of the major uses of TEE in the operating room has been in the preoperative and postoperative assessment of the mitral valve in conjunction with surgery for mitral valve repair. A dramatic increase in the number of attempted and successful surgical reparative procedures on the mitral valve has occurred in the last decade for a number of reasons. First, a considerable body of evidence from animal and human studies has accumulated indicating that patients undergoing mitral valve repair as opposed to replacement emerge with better preserved left ventricular systolic function. The most likely mechanism for this is preserved mitral leaflet/chordae/papillary muscle integrity contributing to a more normal ventricular pumping mechanism. Because the most common cause of early death after valve replacement is low cardiac output from pump failure, mitral valve repair with greater preservation of systolic function has resulted in lower operative mortality than mitral valve replacement. Other reasons for the increasing popularity of mitral repair include a lower incidence of thromboembolism and therefore less need for anticoagulation with repair versus replacement and reduced risk of endocarditis.

Also fueling the trend toward increased repair has been the development of intraoperative echocardiography. Initially epicardial contrast-enhanced echocardiography was used in operative settings followed by color Doppler epicardial echocardiography. Early studies demonstrated the superiority of echocardiographic evaluation of mitral valve integrity to the conventional surgical methods, including fluid filling of the arrested left ventricle, measurement of left atrial V wave height, or digital palpitation of the left atrium for thrills. With the development of TEE and more specifically TEE with color flow capabilities, the intraoperative assessment of valvular repair procedures has been greatly enhanced.

TEE assessment of the mitral valve is useful to the cardiothoracic surgeon both before and after the repair. The preoperative study performed either before the operation in the awake patient operatively or immediately before going on cardiopulmonary bypass can be extremely helpful in providing more precise definition of mitral valvular anatomy. Large series of intraoperative echo in valve repair report findings that altered the planned surgical approach in 15% to 20% of patients. TEE, of course, allows detailed evaluation of mitral leaflet thickening, mobility, and calcification. The presence of myxomatous, redundant tissue can be determined along with definition of leaflet prolapse, inadequate coaptation, or both. Torn chordae are more easily recognized by TEE as well as vegetations and leaflet thickening, mobility, and calcification (Fig. 5-4). Involvement of the mitral subvalvular apparatus, including papillary muscles and chordal structures with thickening or calcification, is readily assessed. All of this information is useful both in determining the feasibility of mitral repair and in planning the exact surgical technique likely to be optimal for the particular valve.

A useful classification of leaflet morphology recognizes three categories of leaflet range of motion: (1) Excessive leaflet motion—seen with prolapsed leaflets as a result of chordal/leaflet/papillary muscle elongation or flail leaflets as a result of ruptured chordae tendineae. These types of abnormalities, especially flail of the middle scallop of the posterior leaflet, have the highest success rate for repair. Techniques employed include quadrilateral resection of the posterior leaflet, chordal shortening, and transfer and creation of chordae. (2) Restricted motion—seen with rheumatic carditis and papillary muscle dysfunction. Mobility of these valves can be increased surgically by commissurotomy, decalcification, and opening of fused chordae. Success rates for these types of repairs are generally lower than for valves exhibiting excessive motion. (3) Normal motion—seen with leaflet perforation and cleft mitral valve. Surgical repair consists of suture closure of the perforation or cleft with insertion of variable amounts of prosthetic material.

Color flow Doppler is used to assess the severity of mitral regurgitation before surgery and contributes to the understanding of the

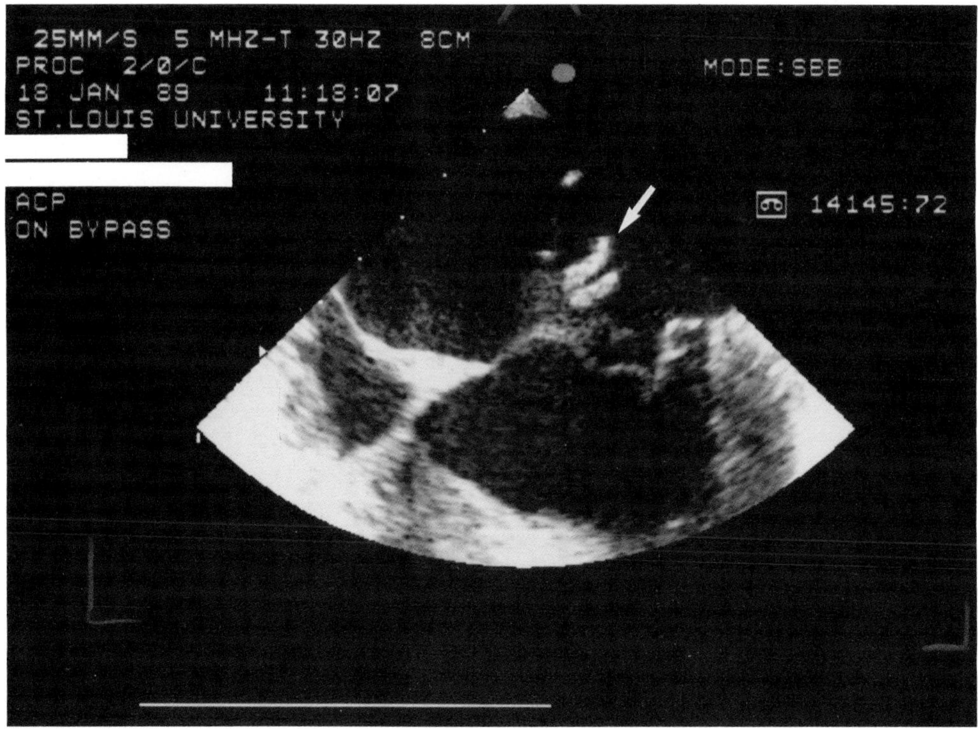

FIGURE 5-4. Flail mitral leaflet with torn chordae (*arrow*) demonstrated by TEE preoperatively.

pathoanatomy of the mitral valve. In general, the color flow jet is directed opposite to the most diseased leaflet. Therefore for posterior flail leaflets, the jet will be directed eccentrically toward the atrial septum and posterior aortic root. For the less commonly encountered anterior flail mitral valve, the jet is directed superolaterally toward the lateral left atrial free wall. We use criteria validated against angiography as described in Chapter 12 to assess the degree of mitral regurgitation.

Following the repair procedure, the valve is reassessed with both complete imaging and color flow Doppler. The optimal time following removal from cardiopulmonary bypass for evaluation varies from patient to patient. It is important to be sure that hemodynamics have returned to optimal conditions for evaluation of the postoperative severity of mitral regurgitation. The left ventricle must be filled optimally with conditions approximating normal hemodynamics. This will generally be more than 10 to 20 minutes after removal from bypass.

Careful attention is paid to the leaflet morphology to check for continued excessive or restricted motion, to exclude suture dehiscence, and to ensure adequate opening. Color Doppler is applied in the four-chamber view to determine the competence of the valve and success

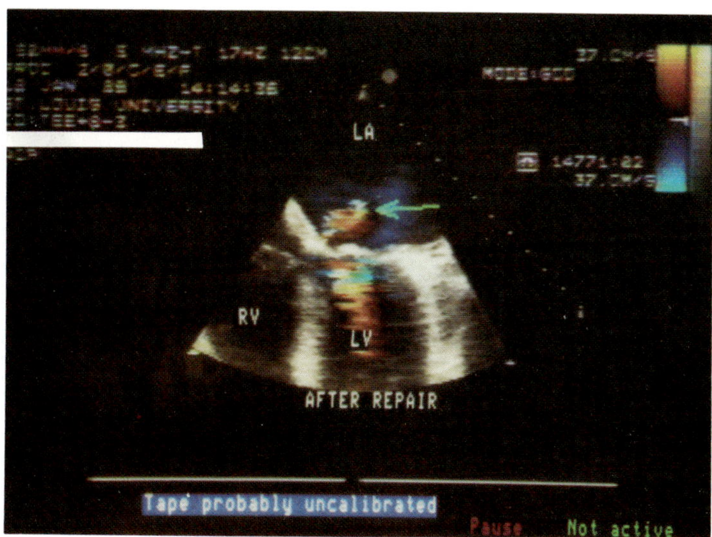

FIGURE 5-5. Mitral valve after repair procedure demonstrating trivial mitral regurgitation.

of repair. A successful repair exhibits color flow jets of mild or trivial severity (Fig. 5-5) with no evidence of significant mitral stenosis. Valves exhibiting more than mild regurgitation may require reoperation. The decision to reoperate is made in consultation with the surgeon and takes into account the following factors: (1) ease of correction of mitral regurgitation (suture dehiscence is easily corrected (Fig. 5-6), continued restriction of rheumatic leaflet more difficult), (2) age of patient, (3) additional procedures (coronary grafting), and (4) severity of mitral regurgitation—clear-cut severe mitral regurgitation will obviously mandate either rerepair or replacement.

The development of systolic anterior motion of the mitral valve has been reported after mitral valve repair. This phenomenon appears especially in patients receiving Carpentier annuloplasty rings. If systolic anterior motion is noted, volume should be infused and pressor support removed if possible to determine the reversibility of the phenomenon. If continuous wave Doppler is available with the TEE probe, the left ventricular outflow tract gradient can be determined. Epicardial echocardiography can also be applied if continuous wave Doppler is not available with the TEE probe. For gradients over 36 mm Hg that do not respond to volume loading or pressor removal, a reoperation is generally advised either to remove the annuloplasty ring or replace the valve. The long-term significance of these abnormalities, however, is not clear.

Sheikh et al. recently reported on the Duke experience with intraoperative TEE in patients undergoing valve surgery (Table 5-1). Prebypass imaging in 154 consecutive patients yielded unsuspected findings that either assisted or changed the planned operation in 29 (19%)

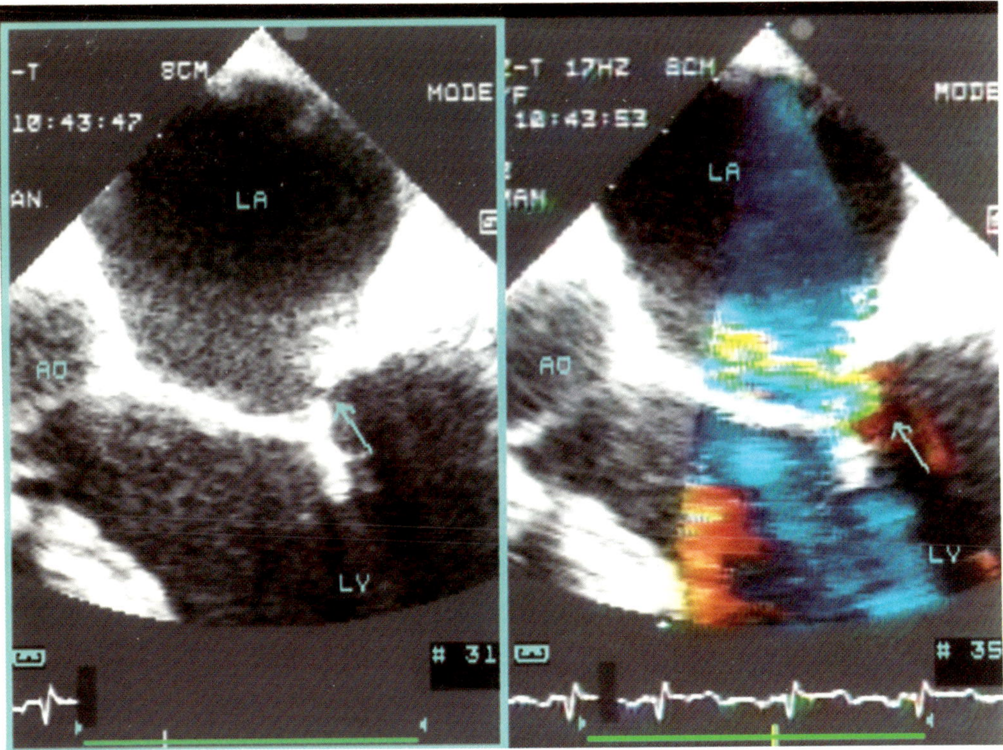

FIGURE 5-6. Dehiscence of suture in posterior leaflet following quadrilateral resection resulting in 3 + mitral regurgitation and need for reoperation.

TABLE 5-1. Utility of TEE in Valve Operations

	Mitral (n = 92)	Aortic (n = 62)
Prebypass		
Modified planned surgery	13 (14)*	2 (3)
Changed planned surgery	10 (11)	4 (6)
Postbypass (valve assessment)		
Encouraged further surgery	10 (11)	0
Postbypass (ventricular assessment)		
Prompted hemodynamic intervention	9 (10)	4 (4)
Total cases useful	34 (37)	9 (15)

* Values in parentheses represent percent.

Modified from Sheikh, K.H., de Bruijn, N.P., Rankin, J.S., et al.: The utility of transesophageal echocardiography and Doppler color flow imaging in patients undergoing cardiac valve surgery. J. Am. Coll. Cardiol., 81:556, 1990.

cases. Postbypass imaging was most useful in patients undergoing mitral valve surgery and identified unsatisfactory results in 10 of 92 cases, resulting in reoperation.

Postbypass TEE imaging also appears useful for predicting postoperative complications. Of seven patients with moderate valve dysfunction following bypass, six had postoperative complications, and three died. Of 23 patients with reduced left ventricular function, 17 had complications and six died.

Marwick et al. reported on the Cleveland Clinic experience with intraoperative echocardiography in 309 patients undergoing mitral repair. A failed repair requiring reoperation was identified in 26 patients: 10 with left ventricular outflow tract obstruction, 10 with incomplete correction, and 6 with suture dehiscence.

Other Intraoperative Uses of TEE

TEE is useful in a variety of other intraoperative situations. Although we do not routinely monitor valve replacement operations, occasionally TEE is valuable in these situations. TEE can identify obstruction to prosthetic valve motion, which may contribute to a patient's inability to be weaned from cardiopulmonary bypass. TEE has also been used to assess the success of tricuspid valve repair operations.

Bibliography

Cahalan, M.K., and Muhiudeen, I.: Intraoperative TEE: Evaluation of left ventricular filling and function, and detection of myocardial ischemia. Am. J. Cardiac Imag., 4:187–191, 1990.

Carpentier, A., Chauvaud, S., Fabianai, J.N., et al.: Reconstructive surgery of the mitral valve incompetence: Ten year appraisal. J. Thorac. Cardiovasc. Surg., 79:338–348, 1980.

Cosgrove, D.M., Chavez, A.M., Gill, C.C., et al.: Mitral valvuloplasty at the Cleveland Clinic Foundation. Clev. Clin. J. Med., 55:37–42, 1988.

Currie, P.J., and Stewart, W.J.: Intraoperative echocardiography in mitral valve repair for mitral regurgitation. Am. J. Cardiac Imag., 4:192–206, 1990.

Czer, L.S., Maurer, G., Bolger, A.F., et al.: Intraoperative evaluation of mitral regurgitation by Doppler color flow mapping. Circulation, 76(suppl III):108–116, 1987.

David, T.E., Uden, D.E., and Strauss, H.D.: The importance of the mitral valve apparatus in left ventricular function after correction of mitral regurgitation. Circulation, 68(suppl II):76–82, 1983.

Goldman, M.E., Fuster, V., Guarino, T., et al.: Intraoperative echocardiography for the evaluation of valvular regurgitation. Experience in 263 patients. Circulation, 74(suppl I):143–149, 1986.

Goldman, M.E., Mora, F., Guarino, T., et al.: Mitral valvuloplasty is superior to valve replacement for preservation of left ventricular function: An intraoperative two-dimensional echocardiographic study. J. Am. Coll. Cardiol., *10*:568–575, 1987.

Harpole, D., Clement, F.M., Quill, T., et al.: Right and left ventricular performance during and after abdominal aortic aneurysm repair. Ann. Surg., *209*:356–362, 1989.

Marwick, T., Currie, P.J., Stewart, W.J., et al.: Echo evaluation of immediate and late failed mitral valve repair [abstract]. J. Am. Coll. Cardiol. *13*:114A, 1989.

Sheikh, K.H., de Bruijn, N.P., Rankin, J.S., et al.: The utility of transesophageal echocardiography and Doppler color flow imaging in patients undergoing cardiac valve surgery. J. Am. Coll. Cardiol., *15*:363, 1990.

Smith, J.S., Cahalan, M.K., Benefiel, D.J., et al.: Intraoperative detection of myocardial ischemia in high risk patients. Electrocardiography versus two dimensional transesophageal echocardiography. Circulation, *72*:1015–1021, 1985.

Stewart, W.J., Currie, P.J., Lytle, B.M., et al.: Intraoperative Doppler color flow mapping for decision making in valve repair for mitral regurgitation: Technique and results in 100 patients. Circulation, *81*:556–566, 1990.

6

Interventional TEE

TEE has been found to be a useful procedure when used in conjunction with invasive intracardiac procedures. These include both applications that are currently useful as part of clinical care and those that have research applications.

Mitral Balloon Valvuloplasty

TEE examination should be performed in all patients in whom a percutaneous mitral balloon valvuloplasty is contemplated. Before valvuloplasty, TEE is performed to assess whether or not a patient is an appropriate candidate for this technique. Information concerning valve mobility, calcification of valve and subvalvular apparatus, and degree of associated mitral insufficiency are all important factors in predicting short-term and long-term outcome following mitral balloon valvuloplasty. The presence of atrial thrombus is believed by many to be a contraindication to percutaneous balloon valvuloplasty because catheter dislodgment of the thrombus may lead to systemic embolization (Fig. 6-1). Transesophageal examination before valvuloplasty is also helpful in demonstrating other associated valvular abnormalities as well as chamber size and ventricular function.

During the procedure, TEE is useful in guiding the catheter across the intra-atrial septum and in positioning the balloon catheter across the stenotic mitral valve (Fig. 6-2). This technique allows for immediate assessment of the results of the valvuloplasty, including the degree of stenosis and insufficiency. In addition, the size of the iatrogenic atrial septal defect (Fig. 6-3), degree of shunting, and complications such as pericardial effusion can be clearly appreciated.

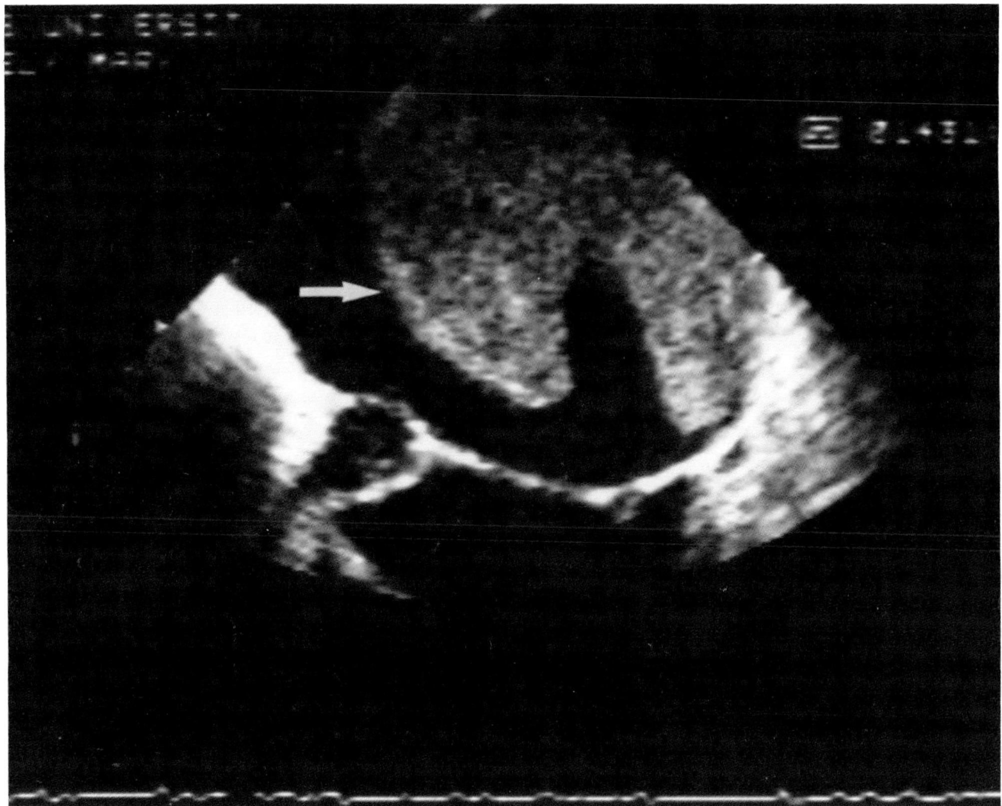

FIGURE 6-1. TEE four-chamber view demonstrating a large left atrial thrombus (*arrow*) in a patient with mitral stenosis who was referred for balloon valvuloplasty. This patient subsequently underwent surgery for mitral valve replacement and thrombectomy.

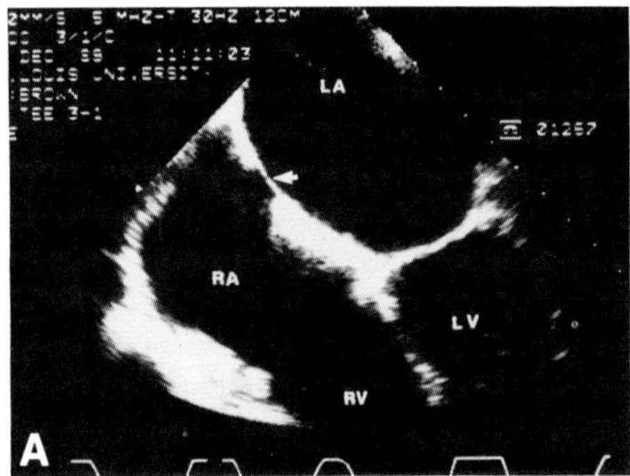
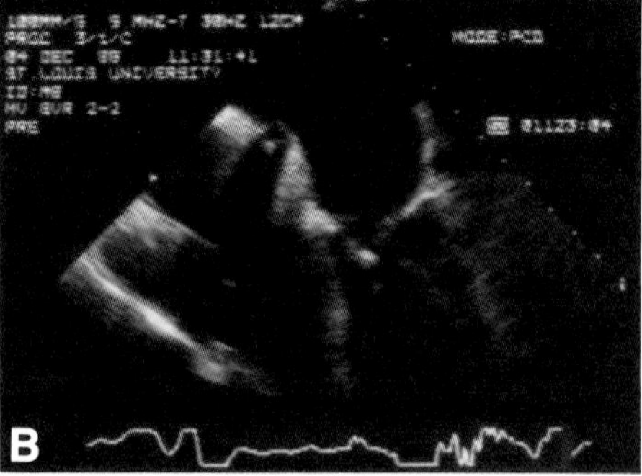

FIGURE 6-2. Echocardiographic four-chamber view demonstrating (A) the fossa ovalis (*arrow*), the preferred site of transseptal crossing; (B) bowing of the intra-atrial septum by the transseptal catheter.

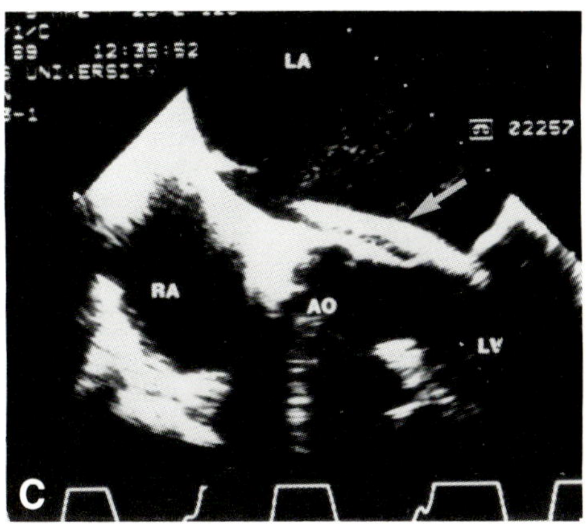

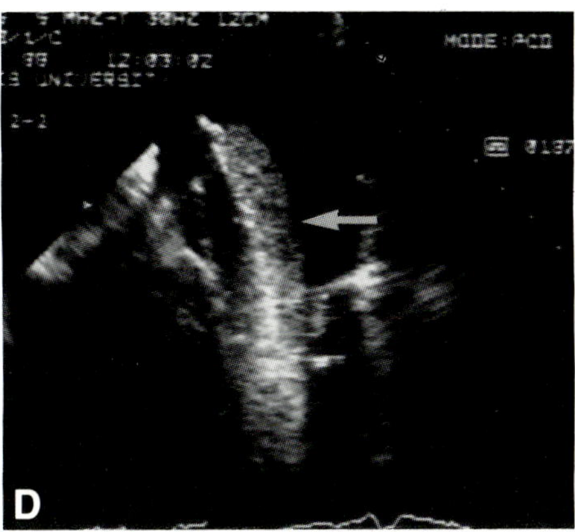

FIGURE 6-2. (*Continued*) (C) positioning of the balloon catheter across the stenotic mitral valve (*arrow*); and (D) fully inflated (*arrow*) balloon catheter.

Atrial Septal Defect Closure

Several investigators have reported on the success of atrial septal defect closure using percutaneous catheter devices. These include both balloon closure for short-term management of interatrial shunting (Fig. 6-4) with a balloon catheter and definitive closure of defects with the "clam shell" type device (Fig. 6-5). TEE is indispensable in assessing the degree of shunting across the defect before closure, positioning the

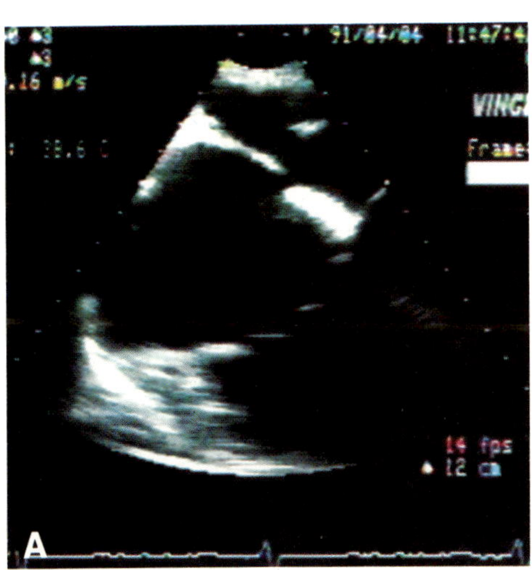

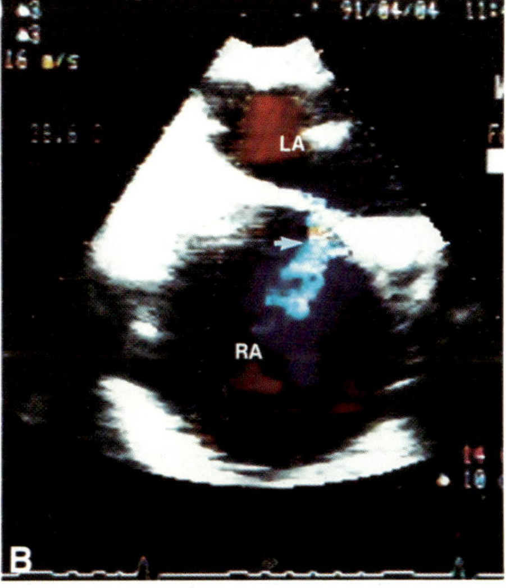

FIGURE 6-3. A 5-mm atrial septal defect is seen (A) with associated left to right shunting (B) following balloon valvuloplasty.

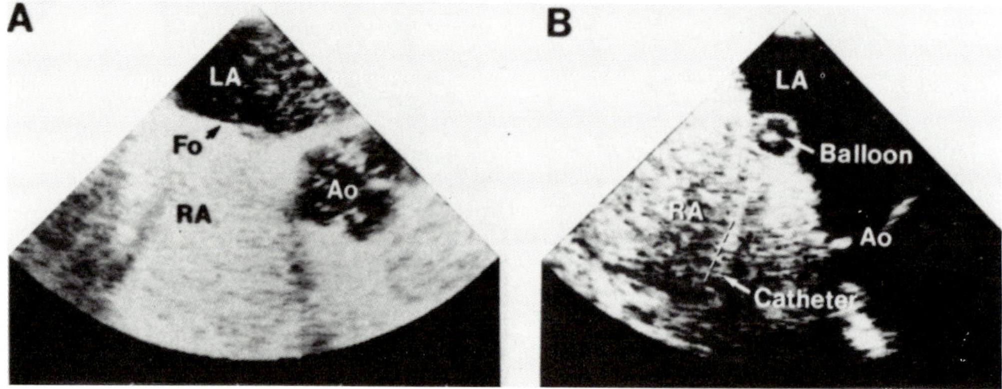

FIGURE 6-4. TEE contrast-enhanced studies demonstrating the degree of shunting across a patent foramen (Fo) (A) before and (B) following balloon catheter closure of the defect. This patient was severely hypoxic as a result of right to left shunting, secondary to elevated right atrial pressure, following a right ventricular myocardial infarction.

catheter or device properly, and assessing the results of closure, usually with an injection of 10 ml of agitated saline.

Ventricular Septal Defect Closure

Recent reports have indicated that TEE guidance may be helpful in percutaneous closure of ventricular septal defects. Positioning of clo-

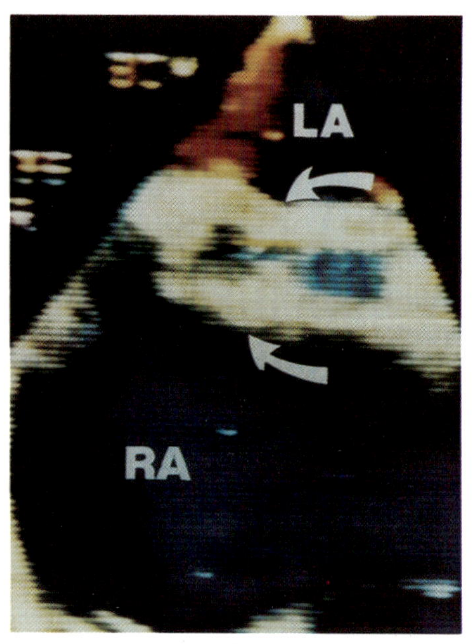

FIGURE 6-5. TEE image demonstrating closure of an atrial septal defect by transcatheter "clam shell" device (*arrows*). From Hellenbrand, W.E., et al.: Transesophageal echocardiographic guidance of transcatheter closure of atrial septal defect. Am. J. Cardiol., *66*:207–213, 1990.

sure device as well as assessment for residual shunt is facilitated by this technique.

Coronary Artery Visualization

Several investigators have examined the ability of TEE to visualize proximal coronary arteries. Success rate for visualization of the left main coronary artery is approximately 90%. Visualization of the proximal circumflex and left anterior descending coronary arteries are in the range of 80 and 70%, respectively (Fig. 6-6). The right coronary artery is somewhat more difficult to examine and is seen well only in approximately 25% of all patients examined. A few investigators have examined the sensitivity of TEE for diagnosing coronary artery stenosis in the proximal coronary segments. Yoshida reported the sensitivity of

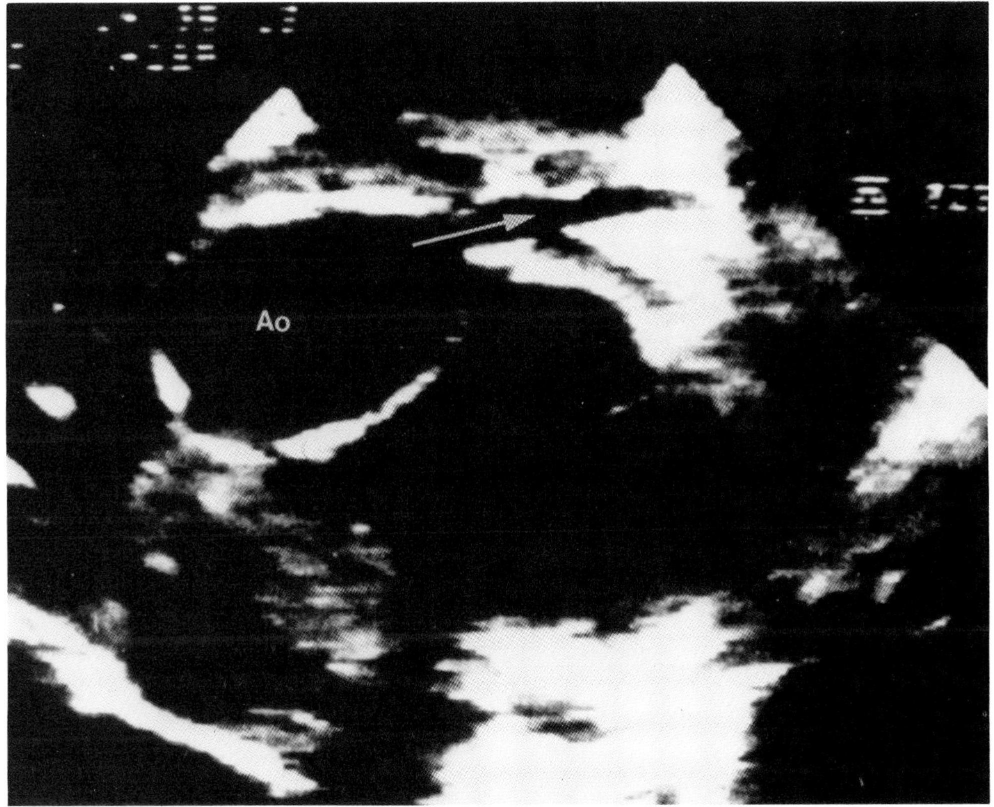

FIGURE 6-6. Basal short-axis view in the upper esophagus demonstrating the origin of left main artery of the aortic root and its bifurcation (*arrow*), with the circumflex artery running roughly parallel to the left main artery in this plane and the anterior artery descending coursing downward.

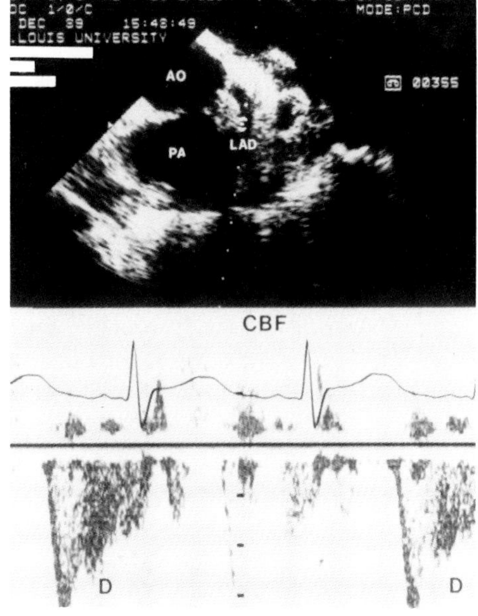

FIGURE 6-7. Pulsed Doppler recording of coronary blood flow (CBF) in the left anterior descending (LAD) coronary artery by TEE.

approximately 75% for the diagnosis of left main stenosis of greater than 50%.

Coronary flow can be assessed by placing the sample volume in the proximal coronary segments (Fig. 6-7). The normal coronary vascular bed has the ability to increase flow severalfold in response to vasodilatation. This coronary flow reserve is impaired in the presence of significant coronary stenoses. Accordingly intracoronary or intravenous injection of coronary vasodilators such as dipyridamole, adenosine, or papaverine can be administered and coronary flow measured both at baseline and after drug administration. The blunting of this so-called hyperemic response may be useful in indicating the presence of significant coronary stenoses downstream. Iliceto et al. have shown these techniques to be applicable when using TEE to measure coronary flow (Fig. 6-8).

Myocardial Perfusion

Both conventional transthoracic echocardiography and TEE have been used during balloon angioplasty to evaluate the effects of ischemia on left ventricular function. The improved visualization of both myocardium and endocardium has allowed a more accurate description of the perfusion distribution of a particular coronary artery. Research applications have included the temporal sequence of events following balloon inflation, such as the association of diastolic ventricular function, systolic wall motion abnormalities, and associated electrocardio-

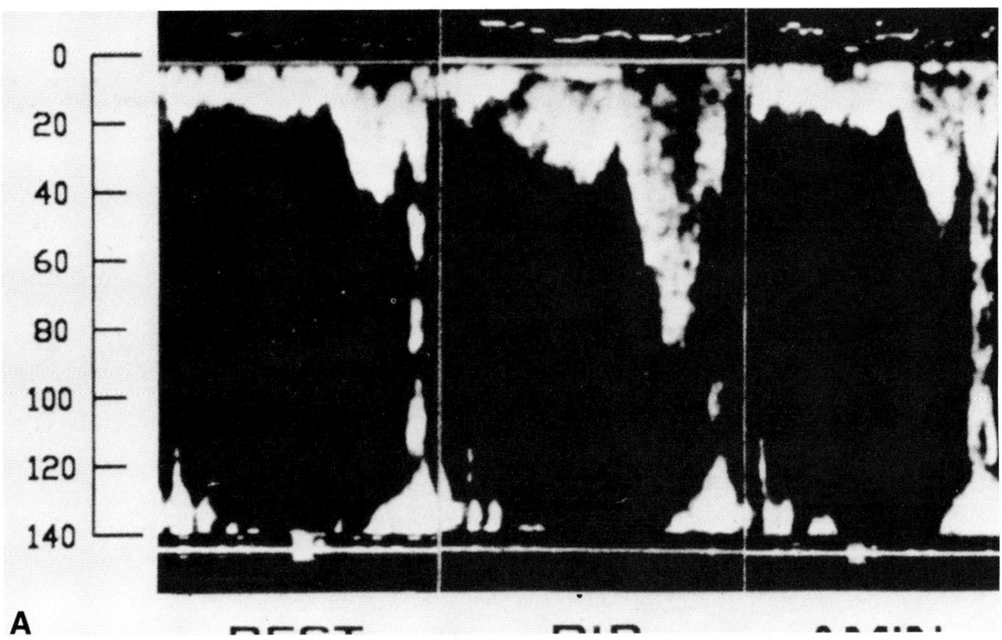

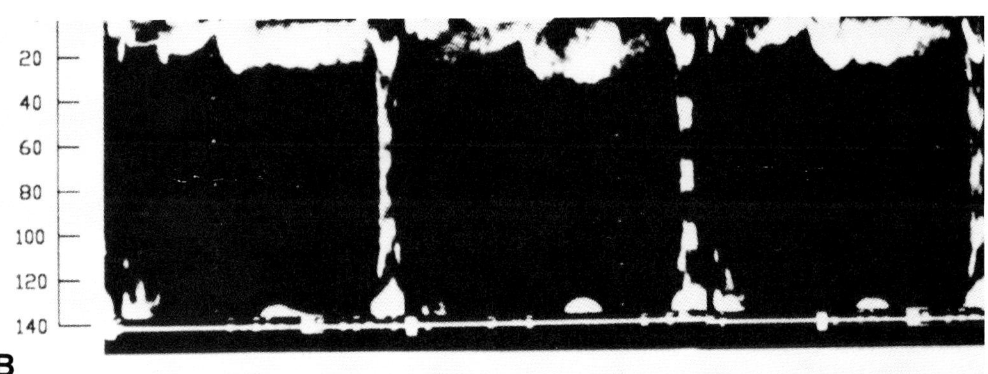

FIGURE 6-8. Coronary blood flow in a normal (A) and stenosed (B) coronary artery after dipyridamole (Dip) and aminophylline (Amin). Note the blunted response to dipyridamole in the stenotic artery. From Iliceto, Sabino, et al.: Transesophageal Doppler echocardiography evaluation of coronary blood flow velocity in baseline conditions and during dipyridamole-induced coronary vasodilation. Circulation, *83*:61–69, 1991.

graphic changes, and the effects of collateral circulation on ischemic segmental dysfunction.

Myocardial perfusion can also be evaluated by assessing the effect on myocardial brightening of intracoronary injections of echo contrast agents. The superior imaging capabilities offered by TEE allow visual or computer-assisted evaluation of myocardial perfusion in the seg-

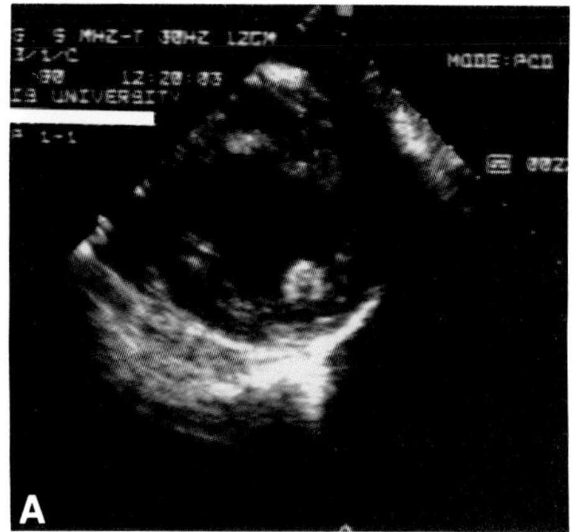 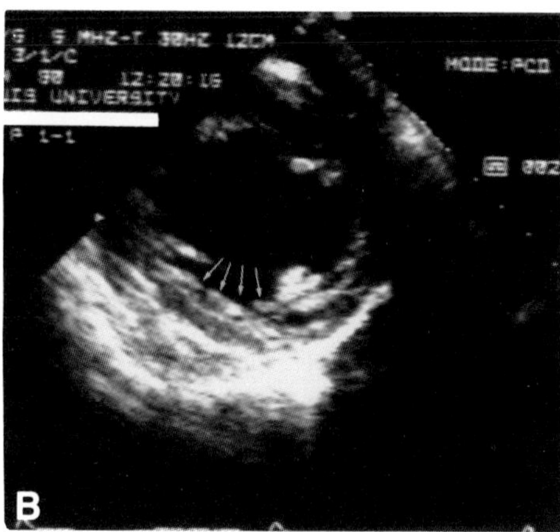

FIGURE 6-9. Echocardiographic short-axis views before (A) and following (B) injection of sonicated echo contrast agent into the left coronary artery. Note the brightening (*arrows*) in the perfusion bed of this vessel.

ments supplied by the coronary artery in question (Fig. 6-9). Although still in the research stage, various echocardiographic contrast agents are being evaluated with these properties.

Heart Biopsy

Several centers perform transvenous right ventricular endocardial biopsy using ultrasound imaging of the forceps in the right atria and right ventricle. Recent reports suggest that TEE may be helpful in cases in which transthoracic echocardiography is technically suboptimal (Fig. 6-10).

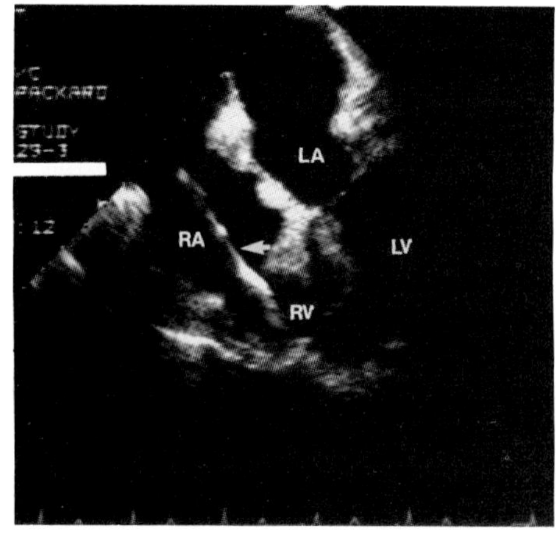

FIGURE 6-10. TEE four-chamber view demonstrating the position of the bioptone (*arrow*) in the right ventricle (RV) during RV endocardial biopsy.

Pericardial Tamponade

TEE has been reported to be useful in a variety of different situations in the cardiac catheterization laboratory. In the occasional patient in whom TEE fails to provide technically satisfactory images, TEE has demonstrated the presence of pericardial effusion and tamponade complicating a procedure and has been useful in guiding therapeutic diagnostic pericardiocentesis.

Bibliography

Ballal, R.S., Mahan, E.F., Nanda, N.C., and Dean, L.S.: Utility of transesophageal echocardiography in interatrial septal puncture during percutaneous mitral balloon commissurotomy. Am. J. Cardiol., 66:230–232, 1990.

Chan, K.L., Marquis, J.F., Ascah, C., et al.: Role of transesophageal echocardiography in percutaneous balloon mitral valvuloplasty. Echocardiography, 7:115–123, 1990.

Hellenbrand, W.E., Fahey, J.T., McGowan, F.X., et al.: Transesophageal echocardiographic guidance of transcatheter closure of atrial septal defect. Am. J. Cardiol., 66:207–213, 1990.

Iliceto, S., Marangelli, V., Memmola, C., and Rizzon, P.: Transesophageal Doppler echocardiography evaluation of coronary blood flow velocity in baseline conditions and during dipyridamole-induced coronary vasodilation. Circulation, 83:61–69, 1991.

Jaarsma, W., Visser, C.A., Suttorp, M.J., et al.: Transesophageal echocardiography during percutaneous balloon mitral valvuloplasty. J. Am. Soc. Echo., 3:384–391, 1990.

Koolen, J.J., Visser, C.A., David, G.K., et al.: Transesophageal echocardiographic assessment of systolic and diastolic dysfunction during percutaneous transluminal coronary angioplasty. J. Am. Soc. Echo., 3:374–383, 1990.

Pearce, F.B., Sheikh, K.H., deBruijn, N.P., and Kisslo, J.: Imaging of the coronary arteries by transesophageal echocardiography. J. Am. Soc. Echo., 2:276–283, 1989.

Yamagishi, M., Yasu, T., Ohara, K., et al.: Detection of coronary blood flow associated with left main coronary artery stenosis by transesophageal Doppler color flow echocardiography. J. Am. Coll. Cardiol., 17:87–93, 1991.

Yoshida, K., Yoshikawa, J., Hozumi, T., et al.: Detection of left main coronary artery stenosis by transesophageal color Doppler and two-dimensional echocardiography. Circulation, 81:1271–1276, 1990.

7

Aortic Dissection

TEE represents a major advance in the diagnosis and understanding of pathology of the thoracic aorta. The proximity of the esophagus to the descending aorta and aortic arch has dramatically altered the role of echocardiography in the evaluation of aortic aneurysm and dissection. In many centers worldwide, TEE is the diagnostic modality of choice for acute aortic dissection.

Aortic Dissection

Aortic dissection is a cardiovascular emergency occurring at a rate of approximately 2000 cases per year in the United States. The mortality rate has been reported to be as high as 80% within 2 weeks, and 40% of patients do not survive until diagnosis. The DeBakey classification (Fig. 7-1) is widely used and recognizes three types of dissection. Types I and II involve the proximal aorta and are also classified as *proximal*, whereas type III involves only the descending (extrapericardial) aorta and has been termed *distal*. The proximal types of dissection are the most dangerous, with potential for rupture into the pericardial sac, followed by cardiac tamponade, dissection into the coronaries with

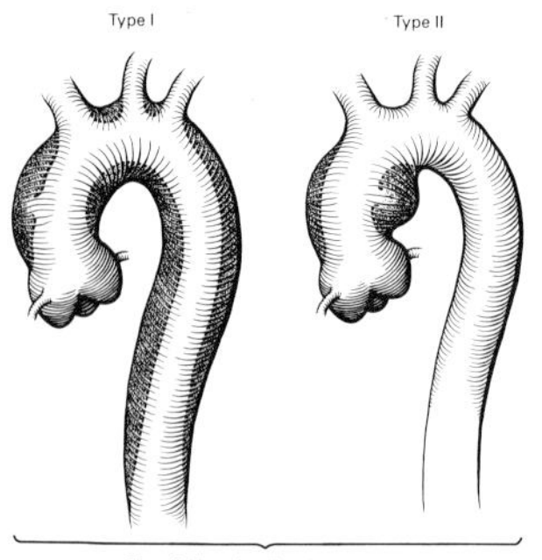

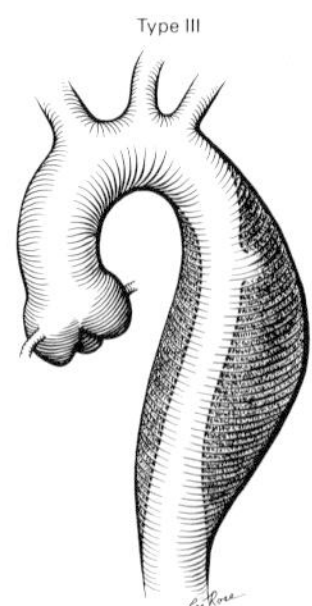

FIGURE 7-1. DeBakey classification of aortic dissection. (From Massumi, A.: Clinical recognition of aortic dissection. Texas Heart Inst J 17:254–256, 1990.)

myocardial infarction, involvement of the aortic annulus or leaflets with aortic regurgitation, and involvement of the great vessels with neurologic consequences. The consensus of opinion is that proximal dissections require prompt surgical correction, whereas medical therapy offers a relative advantage over surgery in most cases of uncomplicated acute distal dissection.

Diagnostic Imaging and Aortic Dissection

Because of the need for prompt and accurate identification and classification of aortic dissection, many different imaging modalities have been advocated, including two-dimensional echocardiography. Matthew and Nanda in 1984 reported using multiple transducer positions with surface echocardiography, including precordial, subcostal, suprasternal, supraclavicular, right parasternal, infraclavicular, and abdominal to reconstruct the entire aorta in 10 patients with aortic aneurysm and 10 with aortic dissection proved by angiography or surgery. Using this technique, they reported complete accuracy in diagnosing aneurysmal segments and differentiating dissection from nondissection. Granato et al. reported a 100% sensitivity and 88% specificity for surface echocardiography in 56 consecutive patients with aortic dissection.

Although visualization of the proximal portions of the ascending aorta is usually possible from the parasternal windows and the aortic arch can be reasonably imaged from the suprasternal notch window, the descending aorta, especially in its thoracic portion, is difficult to assess by routine ultrasonography. In addition, obesity and emphysema frequently complicate the surface examination and compromise diagnostic accuracy. Thus unfortunately in day-to-day clinical practice, this type of accuracy with surface echocardiography is not generally realized, and most centers rely on either computed tomography or contrast angiography for diagnosis of aortic dissection.

TEE Examination of the Aorta

The proximity of the descending aorta to the esophagus throughout its thoracic extent makes TEE ideal for assessing this vessel for dilatation, dissection, and luminal irregularities. Single-plane TEE also yields excellent images of the aortic root from the level of the semilunar valves to the pulmonary artery level. In addition, the distal two thirds of the aortic arch with great vessels is extremely well visualized by TEE.

Evaluation of the aorta is best done in a systematic fashion. The TEE probe is advanced to the level of the left atrium/aortic valve (usually 25 to 30 cm). Flexion of the probe at this level will usually allow visualization of the aortic valve and proximal aortic root in cross-section. A careful search should be made for proximal dissection flaps. These will appear as prominent, highly mobile echoes extending across the lumen of the proximal aorta (Fig. 7-2). In addition, the presence and severity of any associated aortic insufficiency should be determined. Color flow imaging will demonstrate flow during systole predominantly in the true lumen (Fig. 7-3).

Slow withdrawal of the probe with careful scanning will allow serial assessment of the coronary sinuses with associated coronary ostia, followed by the suprasinus aorta usually up to the level of the pulmonary artery and its bifurcation (Fig. 7-4). The aorta at this level is usually the size of the pulmonary artery, and on-screen measurements can be performed to measure the diameter. Further withdrawal usually results in inadequate images as the air-filled trachea becomes superimposed between the esophagus and the arch portion of the ascending aorta. Longitudinal imaging is helpful for assessing distal aspects of the ascending aorta.

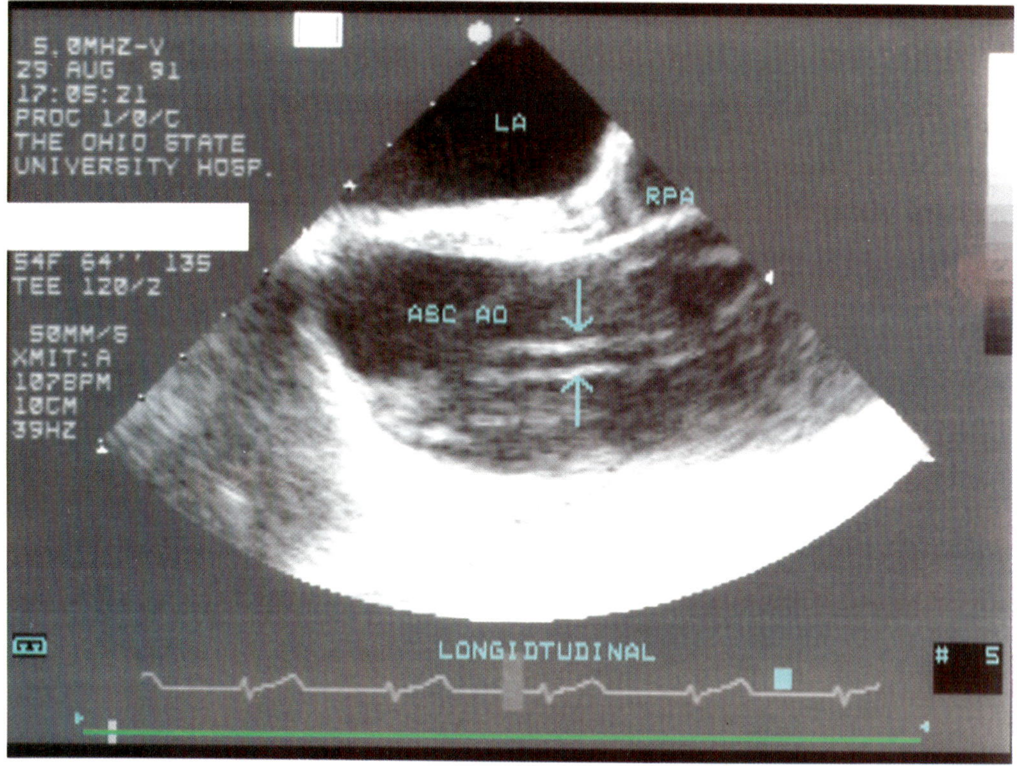

FIGURE 7-2. Longitudinal plane image of ascending aorta (ASC AO) with intimal flap (*arrows*) in a patient with acute type I aortic dissection. Double line is due to reduplication of flap as it recoils. (LA = Left atrium; RPA = right pulmonary artery.)

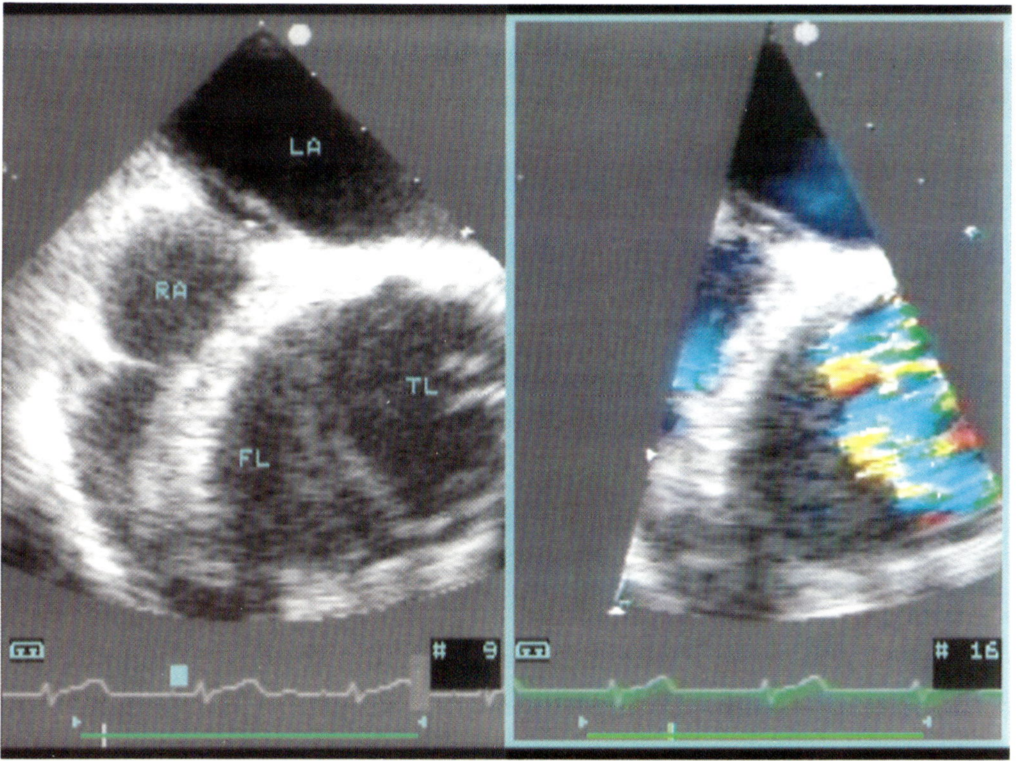

FIGURE 7-3. Transverse plane image of type I aortic dissection with intimal flap separating false lumen (FL) containing spontaneous contrast from true lumen (TL). Color flow superimposition on right demonstrates flow solely in true lumen. (RA = Right atrium; LA = left atrium.)

For assessment of the descending aorta and aortic arch with great vessels, the probe is rotated (usually counterclockwise) approximately 120 degrees until the characteristic circular cavity of the descending aorta comes into view. While scanning the descending aorta, we prefer to reduce the depth to the minimum setting possible, usually 4 to 6 cm, to maximize sensitivity to luminal irregularities and dissection flaps. With depth reduction, of course, it is necessary to reduce gain settings and adjust time, gain, compensation (TGC) controls. Following visualization of the descending aorta, the probe is advanced along the length of the descending aorta. This maneuver will require constant rotation of the probe to keep the descending aorta in the center of the screen owing to the rotation of the esophagus in relation to the descending aorta. The descending aorta can usually be visualized several centimeters below the diaphragm to the level of the proximal abdominal aorta. The probe should then be slowly withdrawn with gentle flexion applied to maximize esophageal/descending aorta contact back up to the level of the arch. During scanning of the descending aorta, it

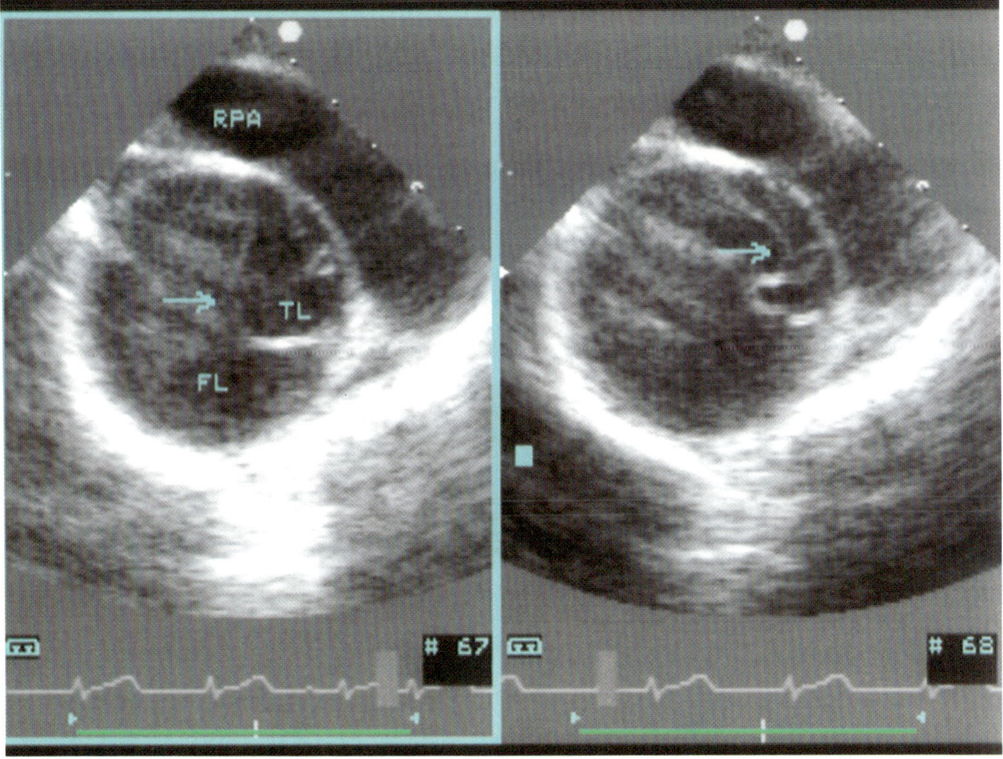

FIGURE 7-4. Transverse plan image at level of pulmonary artery in type I aortic dissection. Systolic frame on left demonstrates expansion of true lumen (TL), whereas diastolic frame on right shows collapse of intimal flap (*arrow*).

is important to monitor the distance of the tip from the incisors to record the location of any pathology noted.

Scanning of the aortic arch and great vessels requires gentle clockwise rotation with an increase in the depth setting. Patients frequently will experience discomfort with the probe at this level in the pharynx, so examinations may be truncated.

TEE Examination in Aortic Dissection

Borner et al. first reported on the use of TEE in aortic dissection in 1984. Subsequent reports from Omoto's group in Japan and Erbel's group in Germany indicated tremendous potential for the technique. The TEE findings in acute aortic dissection are the presence of an intimal flap within the aorta dividing the lumen into true and false lumens. Figure 7-5 demonstrates such an intimal flap in the descending aorta of a patient with acute type III dissection. Such flaps are not subtle, and a characteristic motion is seen in real-time with rapid movement of the flap away from the true lumen during systole and recoil during diastole as the blood flows from true to false lumen. With color flow Doppler superimposed, flow can be noted in the true lumen during systole and in the false lumen during diastole. When flow in the false lumen is reduced by treatment or dilatation of the false lumen, spontaneous echocardiographic contrast may be noted with or without thrombus. Flaps in the ascending aorta may prolapse into left ventricular outflow tract and impede proper closure of the aortic valve, leading to aortic insufficiency.

With careful evaluation of the entire length of the ascending and descending aorta, the length of the dissection and entry and exit tears can be clearly identified. Color flow Doppler is helpful in identifying small entry tears and can be used to time flow from false to true lumen (Fig. 7-6).

Location of the entry tear is crucial in aortic dissection to perform successful surgery and repair the dissection. Hashimoto et al. demonstrated that TEE with color flow Doppler was extremely accurate in localizing this entry tear in comparison with angiography. The entry

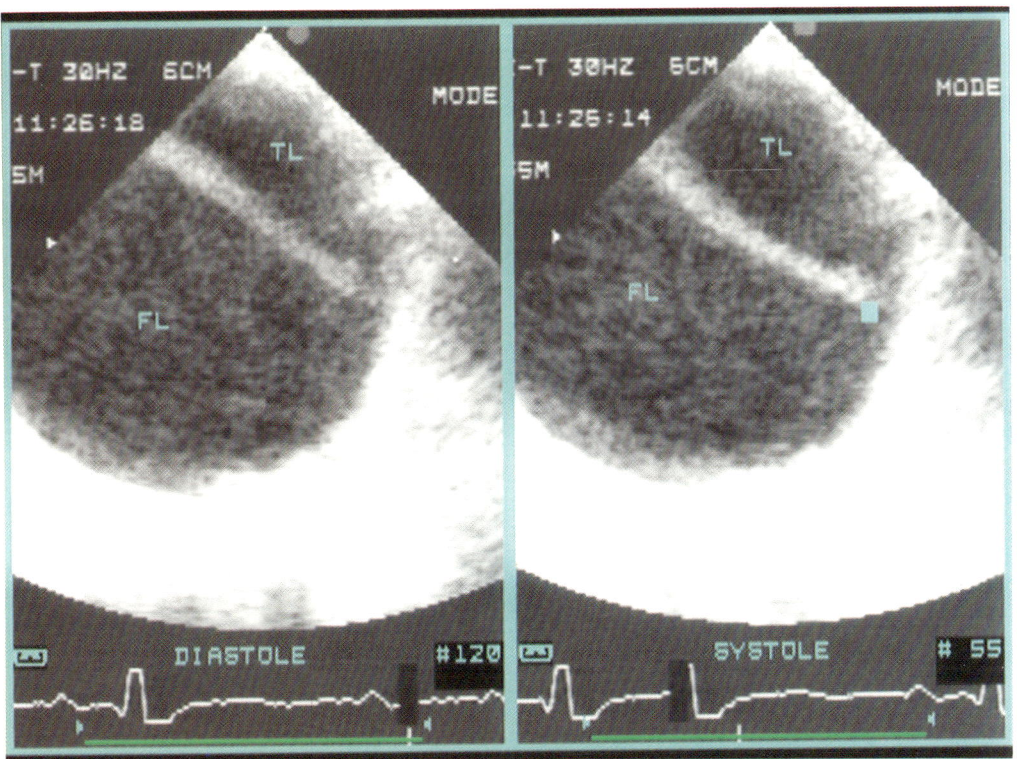

FIGURE 7-5. Transverse plane image of descending aorta in type III aortic dissection. With systole (right), the intimal flap moves out from true lumen (TL) in comparison to diastole (left).

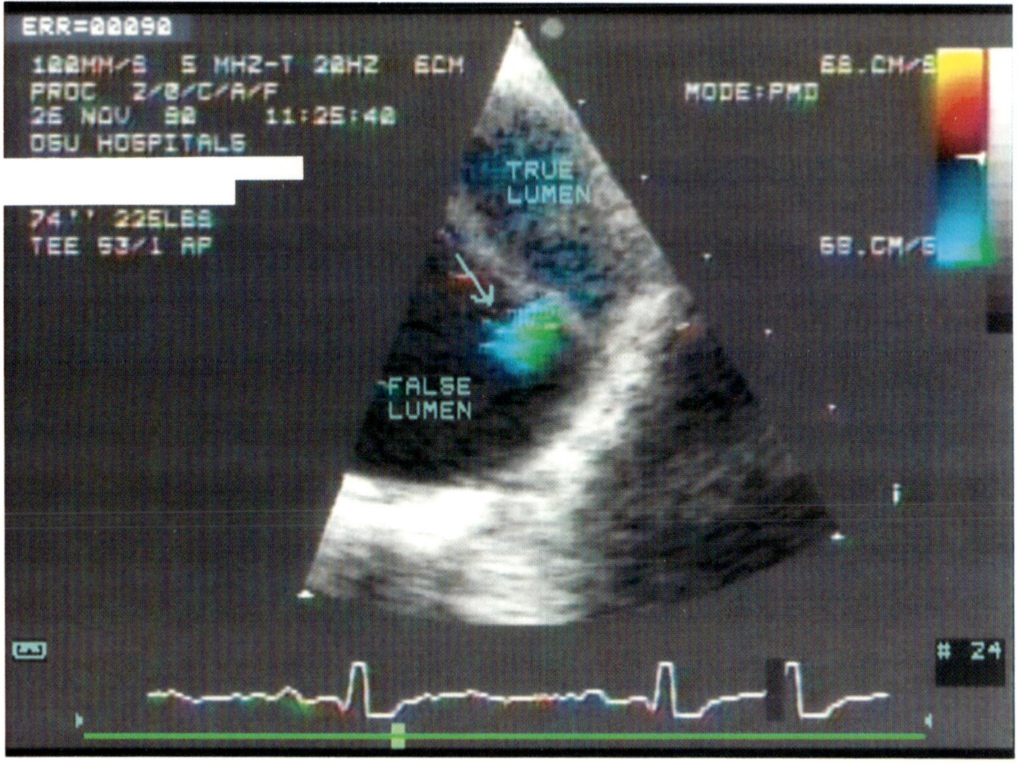

FIGURE 7-6. Color flow imaging in transverse plane of descending aorta demonstrating small entry tear (*arrow*) with color moving from true to false lumen.

site (or re-entry site) is identified as a defect of the intimal flap with a jet of color flow synchronized with the cardiac cycle and moving from true to false lumen (Fig. 7-7). True lumen is usually easy to differentiate from false lumen by the movement of the intimal flap: During systole the flap will move outward from the true lumen toward the false lumen, whereas in diastole the reverse occurs. In addition, if movement of the lumen is reduced, indicating no or little blood flow into the false lumen, the false lumen is usually partially or completely filled by spontaneous contrast, thrombus, or both (Fig. 7-8).

TEE is also useful for evaluation of the aortic valve. The severity and cause of any aortic insufficiency present can be recognized with TEE quite easily. In addition, presence of pericardial effusion is identified with greater accuracy by TEE. Left ventricular function and any other significant valvular disease can also readily be assessed.

It is important to recognize that TEE has a significant blind spot involving the distal portion of the ascending aorta. This blind spot arises as a result of superimposition of the trachea between esophagus and aortic arch (Fig. 7-9). The distal two thirds of the arch can usually be visualized by scanning posteriorly through the superior portion of

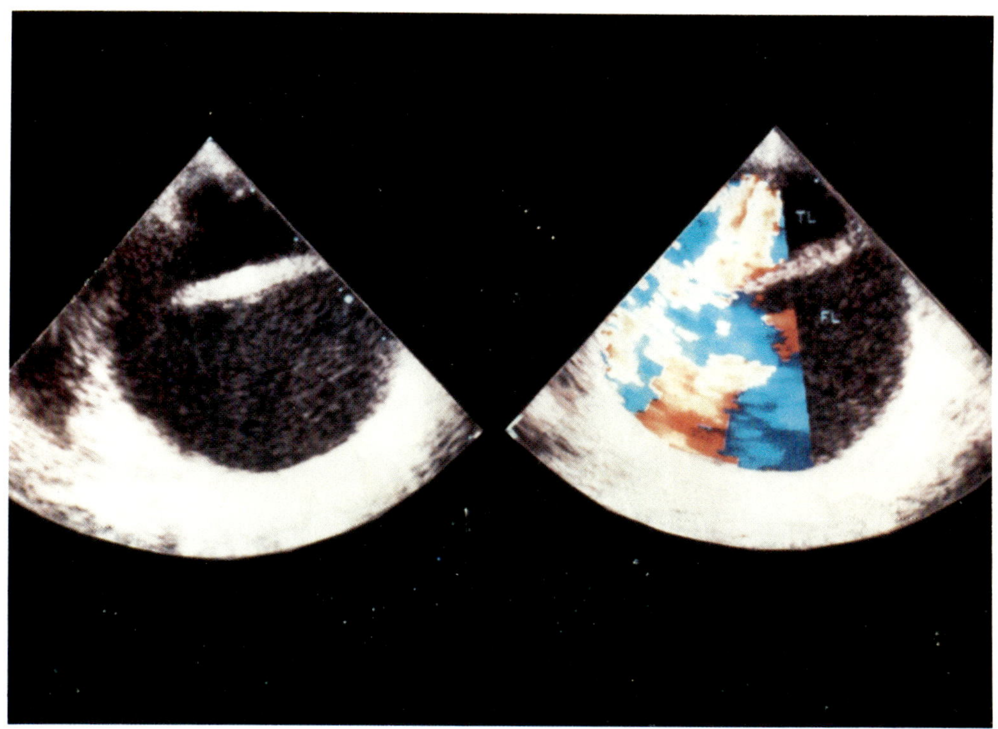

FIGURE 7-7. Large entry tear in descending aorta with color flow superimposed showing large jet moving from true (TL) to false (FL) lumen.

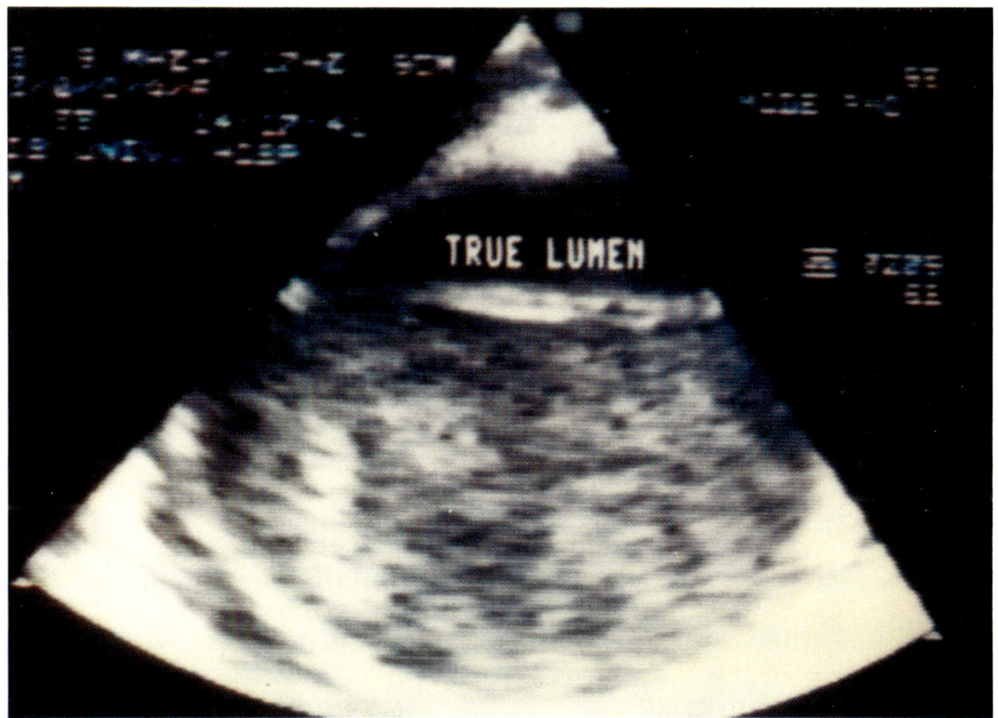

FIGURE 7-8. Type III dissection following treatment demonstrating thrombus in false lumen.

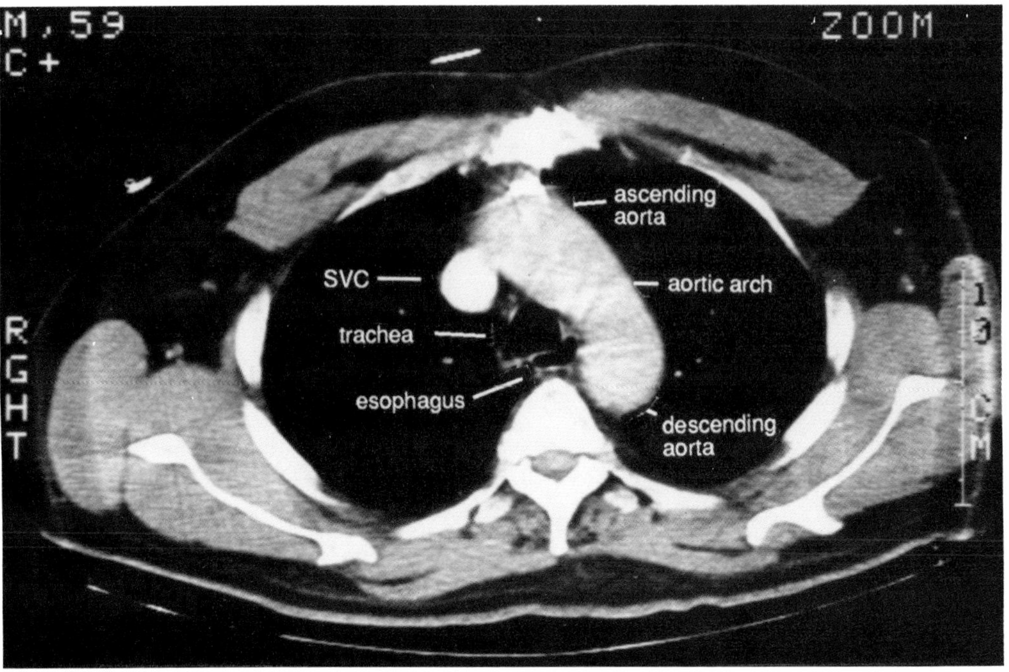

FIGURE 7-9. Computed tomographic scan of thorax at level of aortic arch demonstrating air-filled trachea blocking interrogation of proximal third of arch by probe located in esophagus. (SCV = Superior vena cava.)

the descending aorta (Fig. 7-10). Entry tears and other aortic pathologies including localized type II dissection can be missed in this hidden portion of the ascending aorta. To some extent, this area can be visualized by suprasternal or supraclavicular echocardiography; therefore the ascending aorta should always be examined by the combined technique of transthoracic echocardiography and TEE.

Erbel et al. have reported on the European cooperative study group multicenter trial of echocardiography in aortic dissection. In this study, 164 consecutive patients were examined by transthoracic echocardiography and TEE during 1983 through 1987 at five European centers. Comparison was made to computed tomography or aortic angiography, surgery, or necropsy findings. A diagnosis of aortic dissection was made by echocardiography if two lumens separated by an intimal flap were identified within the aorta. In addition, a completely thrombosed false lumen, central displacement of intimal calcification, or separation of intimal layers from thrombus was also regarded as positive. With echocardiography, only one false-negative result occurred in a patient with type II dissection. Angiography was also negative in this patient, who underwent surgery for severe aortic insufficiency. False-positive diagnoses of type II dissection were made in two patients with aneurysmal proximal aortas as a result of reverberations within the ascending aorta. Importantly, no dissections were detected by computed tomog-

TABLE 7-1. Detection of Aortic Dissection

	Echocardiography (%)	Computed Tomography (%)	Angiography (%)
Group A*			
Sensitivity	98	77	89
Specificity	88	100	87
Group B†			
Sensitivity	100	93	85
Specificity	100	100	97
Group A and B			
Sensitivity	99	83	88
Specificity	98	100	94

* Diagnosis proved at surgery or necropsy.
† Diagnosis proved by at least two methods.

Adapted from Erbel, R., Daniel, W., Visser, C., et al.: Echocardiography in diagnosis of aortic dissection. Lancet, 1:457–459, 1989.

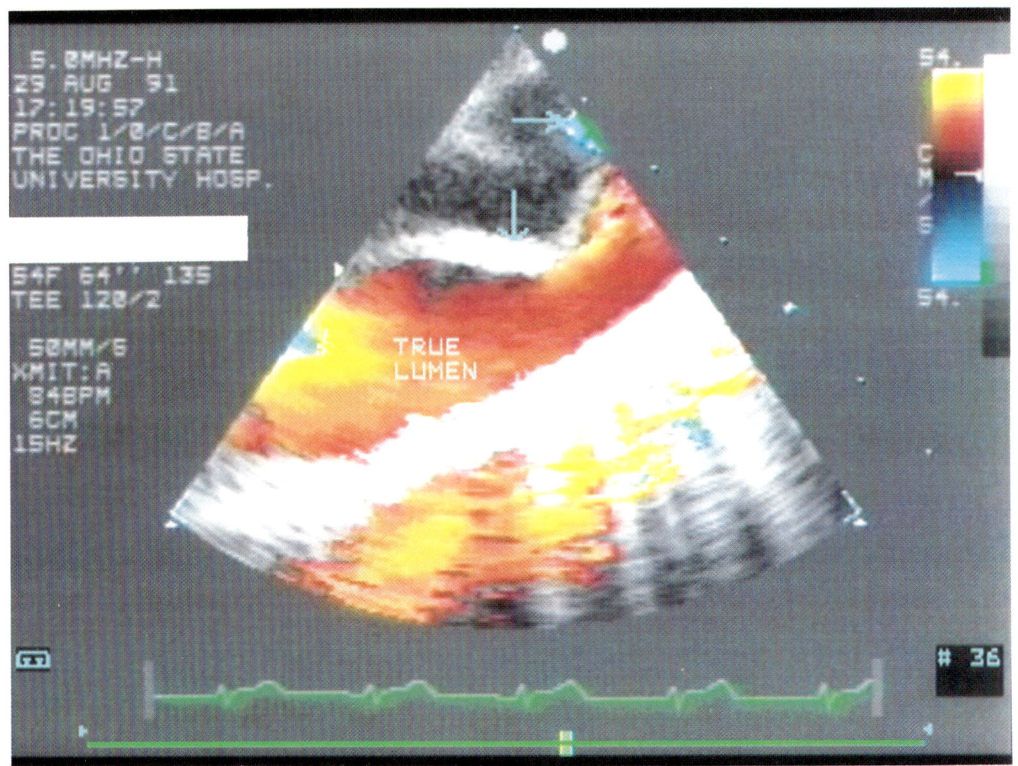

FIGURE 7-10. Transverse plane image of aortic arch (Ao) in patient with type I aortic dissection. Intimal flap is clearly seen (*vertical arrow*). A small blue jet (*horizontal arrow*) indicates the entry tear in the distal portion of the arch.

raphy or angiography if echocardiography was negative. The overall sensitivity and specificity of TEE were 98 and 88%, respectively, for necropsy/surgery documented disease (Table 7-1).

TEE in Follow-up of Aortic Dissection

Survival after surgery for aortic dissection is 57% at 5 years, 32% at 10 years, and 5% at 20 years, with about 30% of late death as a result of aneurysmal rupture. Long-term survival of treated aortic dissection approaches 60% at 10 years. As many as 40% of late deaths are clearly related to complications of the dissection. Reoperations for such late complications have been reported as 13% at 5 years and 23% at 10 years. DeBakey has reported that 29% of all late deaths are caused by late development of aneurysm followed by rupture.

For these reasons, close monitoring of patients with treated aortic dissection is recommended. De Sanctis et al. advise routine chest x-ray films every 3 months for the first year of follow-up and semiannually thereafter. Semiannual computed tomographic scans have been recommended in patients at particularly high risk of aneurysm formation, such as patients with Marfan's syndrome.

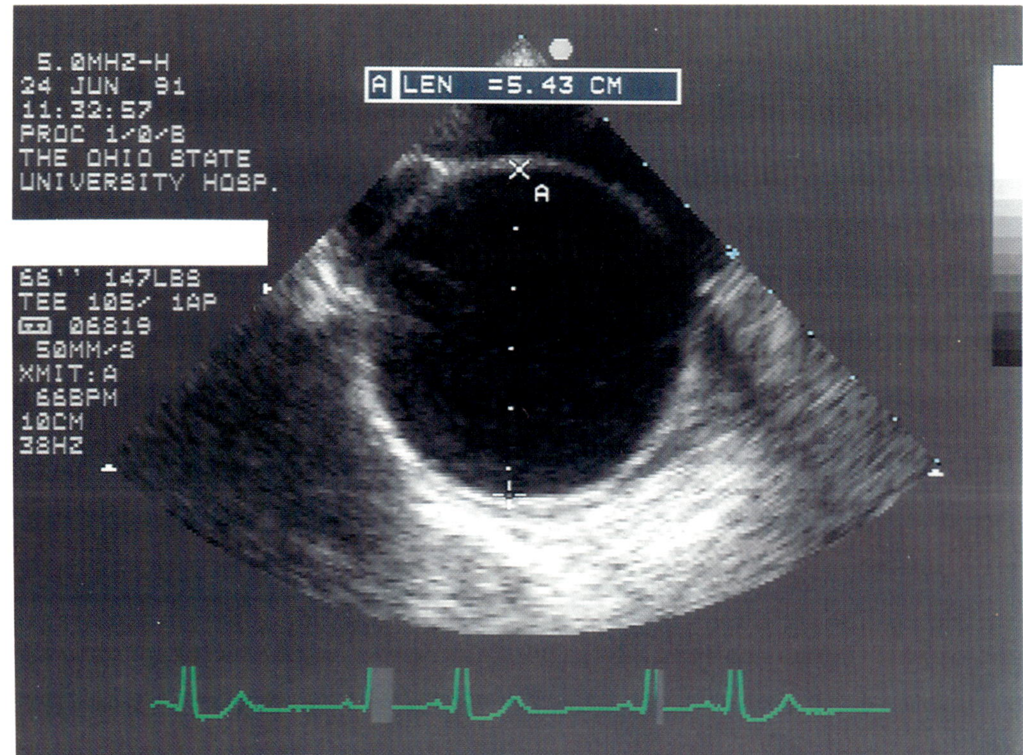

FIGURE 7-11. Transverse plane image of aortic aneurysm at level of pulmonary artery.

TEE would appear to offer an ideal noninvasive technique for the follow-up of treated aortic dissection. It provides excellent information on the late course of the false lumen and aortic size and uses no ionizing radiation. TEE seems to be ideally suited for the follow-up of patients with aortic dissection because of its relatively noninvasive nature and ability to monitor size, thrombus formation, and flow patterns in the false lumen. Mohr-Kahaly studied 18 patients with treated acute aortic dissection and showed a persistence of the false lumen in five of seven after surgery and nine of 11 after medical treatment. Flow within the false lumen was detected in 14 patients. Additional information, including the detection of flow characteristics, extension of dissection, localized dilatation of the aorta, mediastinal hematoma, and aortic regurgitation, was obtained by TEE.

Aortic Aneurysm

Both saccular and fusiform aneurysms of the thoracic aorta have been identified with TEE. In comparison to more established techniques such as computed tomography and angiography, TEE appears at least as accurate in identifying size and location of aneurysm (Figs. 7-11 and 7-12). In one study of 15 patients with thoracic aortic aneurysm, TEE

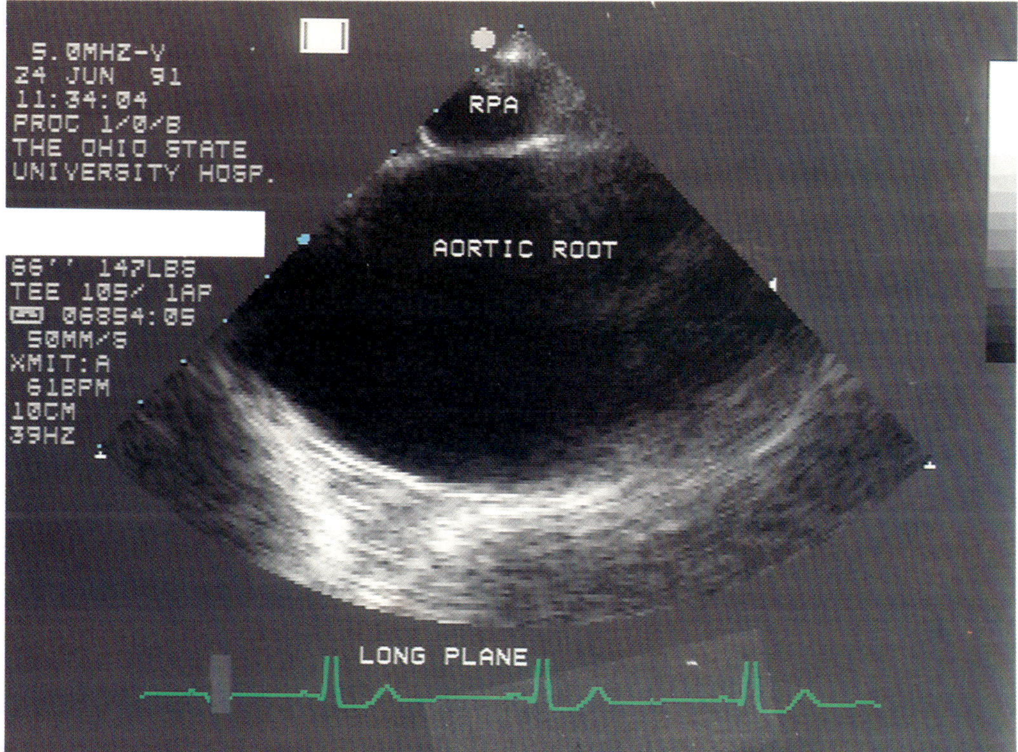

FIGURE 7-12. Longitudinal plane image of ascending aortic aneurysm.

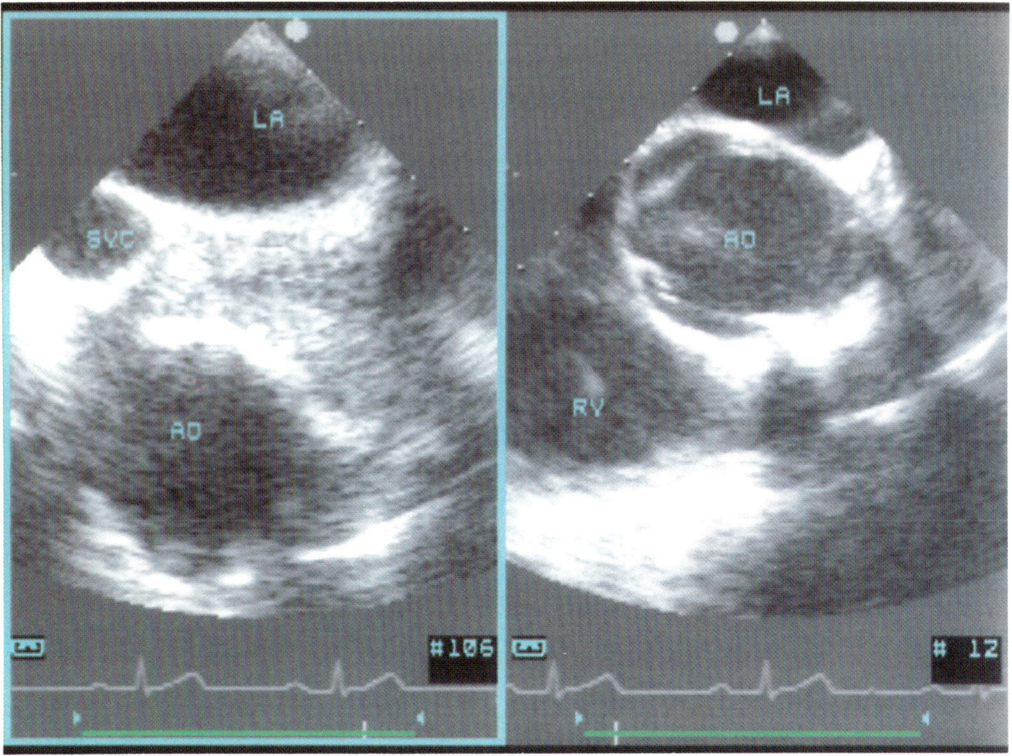

FIGURE 7-13. Transverse scan of ascending aorta in a patient 6 months after repair of ruptured ascending aortic aneurysm. On left at the level of the superior vena cava (SVC), a large hematoma can be seen between the left atrium (LA) and the aortic graft (Ao). On the right, transverse imaging at the level of the aortic valve (Ao) demonstrates dilation of the native aortic root. (RV = Right ventricle.)

made the correct diagnosis in all 15. In contrast, with computed tomography, aneurysms were missed. In one patient, both computed tomography and contrast angiography incorrectly diagnosed aortic dissection in a patient with aneurysm containing thrombus. The distinction between intimal calcifications in an atherosclerotic aorta, calcification on the surface of a thrombus in a fusiform aneurysm, and a thrombosed false lumen of a dissection can usually be made by TEE but is difficult by other modalities.

Following surgery for aortic aneurysm or dissection rupture, large amounts of hematoma will persist in the spaces around the aortic graft (Fig. 7-13). It is important to recognize this as a normal appearance postoperatively. Because the amount of such hematoma varies from patient to patient, TEE examinations postoperatively are important to establish a baseline for subsequent evaluations.

Aortic Ulcer and Atheroma

Atheromatous disease of the aorta is a common but generally asymptomatic process noted with aging. Occasionally embolization from an ulcerated atheroma or overlying thrombus may result in cerebrovascular or peripheral vascular occlusion. Such ulceration is usually confined to the intimal layer of the aorta. These ulcerated plaques are easily recognized by TEE examination because they result in marked luminal irregularity of the descending aorta. Occasionally overlying thrombus can be identified.

Ulceration of the atheromatous plaque may penetrate deeply into the aortic wall. When the ulcer extends into the media, several potential complications may occur. A medial hematoma or localized dissection may be the result. Localization of the dissection is more likely if there is associated medial fibrosis and atrophy limiting propagation through the plane of cleavage. This ulcer may then penetrate locally through the aortic wall to form a pseudoaneurysm.

Clinically the penetrating aortic ulcer may mimic aortic dissection in its presentation. Patients are usually elderly with a history of severe

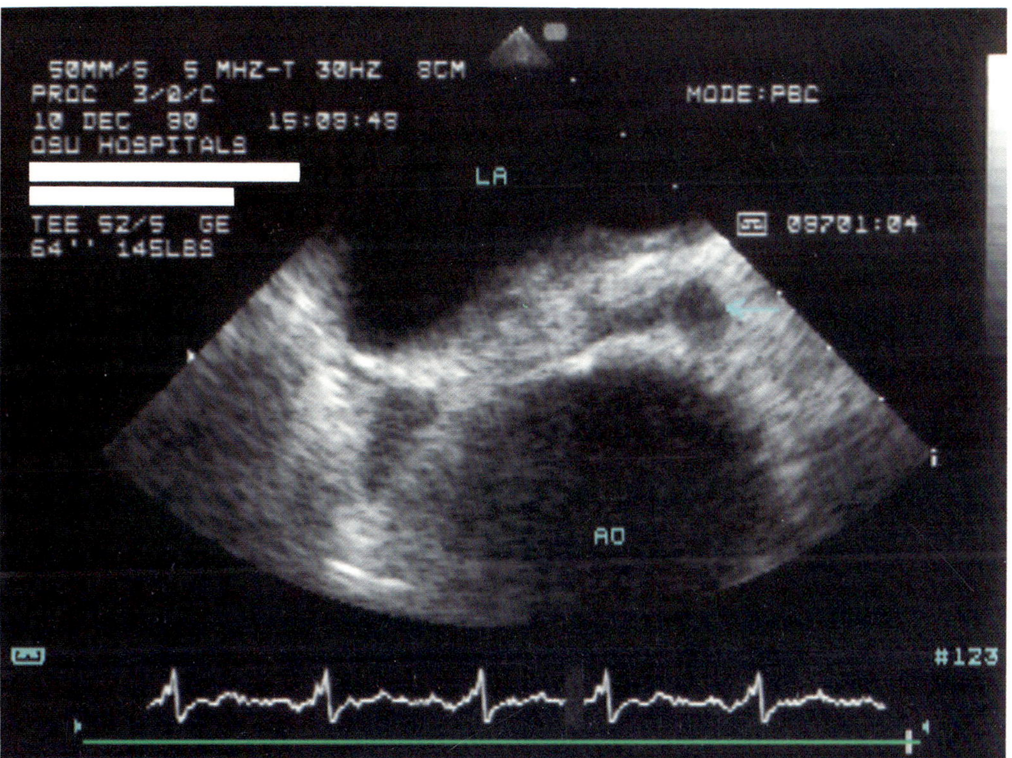

FIGURE 7-14. Intimal hematoma (*arrow*); see text for description.

hypertension and atherosclerosis and develop sudden severe chest or back pain. Diagnosis has in the past been made by contrast-enhanced angiography, computed tomography, or magnetic resonance imaging. Cooke et al. recommended an aggressive surgical approach to this entity following medical treatment with beta-blockade.

There are no reports of surface echocardiography in the diagnosis of aortic ulcer. We have found, however, TEE examination to be useful in the diagnosis of this entity. Figure 7-14 is from a patient who presented with severe chest pain with radiation to the back. Examination by computed tomography demonstrated thickening of the wall of the ascending aorta without an intimal flap. TEE examination was performed to delineate further the pathology in the ascending aorta. An intramural hematoma was discovered but no intimal flap. The patient was treated medically. Two days later, the patient developed more pain, and a contrast-enhanced angiogram revealed an aortic ulcer in the ascending aorta. Repeated TEE examination demonstrated an intimal rupture in the area of previous hematoma (Fig. 7-15). This case demonstrates the utility of TEE examination in repeat examination and following the natural history of aortic pathology.

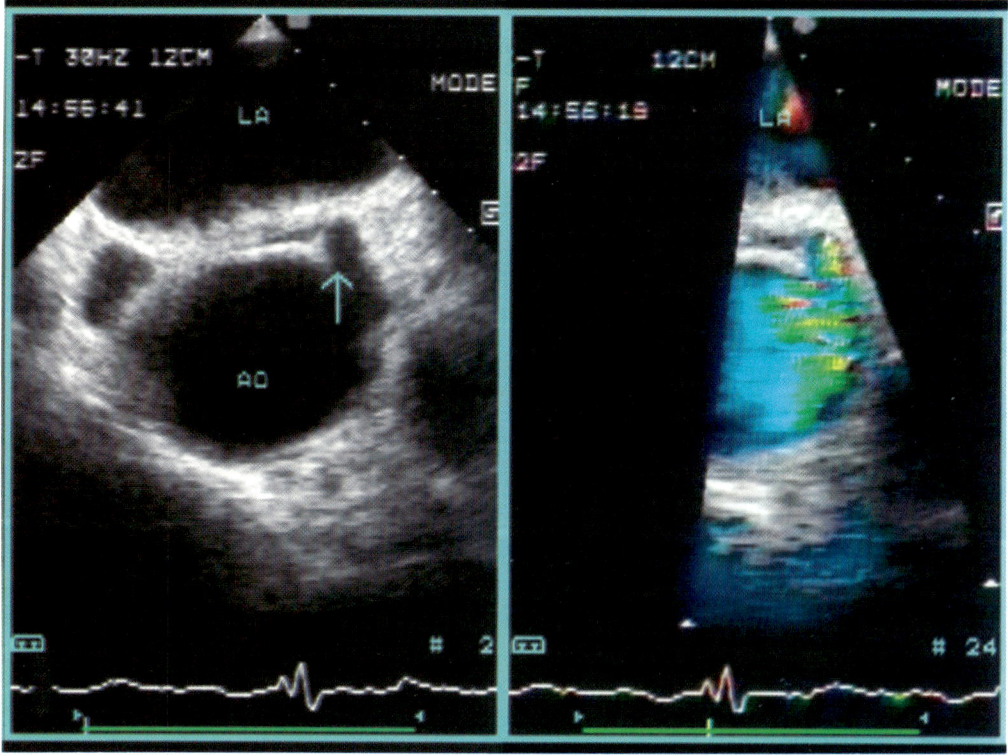

FIGURE 7-15. Aortic ulcer (*arrow*). Note color flow into opening (right).

Bibliography

Borner, N., Erbel, R., Braun, B., et al.: Diagnosis of aortic dissection by transesophageal echocardiography. Am. J. Cardiol., 54:1157–1158, 1984.

Cooke, J.P., Kazmier, F.J., and Orszulak, T.A.: The penetrating aortic ulcer: Pathologic manifestations, diagnosis, and management. Mayo Clin. Proc., 63:718–725, 1988.

DeBakey, M.E., McCollum, C.H., Crawford, E.S., et al.: Dissection and dissecting aneurysms of the aorta: Twenty-year follow-up of five hundred twenty-seven patients treated surgically. Surgery, 92:1118–1134, 1982.

De Sanctis, R.W., Doroghazi, R.M., Austen, G., and Buckley, M.J.: Aortic dissection. N. Engl. J. Med., 317:1060–1068, 1987.

Doroghazi, R.M., Slater, E.E., DeSanctis, R.W., et al.: Long-term survival of patients with treated aortic dissection. J. Am. Coll. Cardiol., 3:1026–1034, 1984.

Erbel, R., Borner, N., Steller, D., et al.: Detection of aortic dissection by transesophageal echocardiography. Br. Heart J., 58:45–81, 1987.

Erbel, R., Daniel, W., Visser, C., et al.: Echocardiography in diagnosis of aortic dissection. Lancet, 1:457–460, 1989.

Erbel, R., Mohr-Kahaly, S., Brunier, J., et al.: Stellenwert der transthorakalen und transosophagealen Echokardiographie in der praoperativen Diagnostik der Aortendissektion. Thorac. Cardiovasc. Surg., 1(suppl1):23, 1987.

Granato, J.E., Dee, P., and Gibson, R.S.: Utility of two-dimensional echocardiography in suspected ascending aortic dissection. Am. J. Cardiol., 56:123–129, 1985.

Hashimoto, S., Kumada, T., Osakada, G., et al.: Assessment of transesophageal Doppler echography in dissecting aortic aneurysm. J. Am. Coll. Cardiol., 14:1253–1262, 1989.

Hashimoto, S., Toshiaki, K., Osakada, G., et al.: Detection of the entry site in dissecting aortic aneurysm using transesophageal Doppler ultrasonography. Am. J. Cardiac Imag., 3:45–52, 1989.

Haverich, A., Miller, D.C., Scott, W.C., et al.: Acute and chronic aortic dissections—determinants of long-term outcome for operative survivors. Circulation, 72(suppl II):II–22–34, 1985.

Mohr-Kahaly, S., Erbel, R., Borner, N., et al.: Kombination von Farb-Doppler und transosophagealer Echokardiographie in der Notfalldiagnostik bei Aortendissektionen vom Typ. I. Z. Kardiol., 75:616–620, 1986.

Mohr-Kahaly, S., Erbel, R., Rennollet, H., et al.: Ambulatory follow-up of aortic dissection by transesophageal two-dimensional and color-coded Doppler echocardiography. Circulation, 80:24–33, 1989.

Takamoto, S., Kyo, S., Matsumara, M., et al.: Total visualization of thoracic dissecting aortic aneurysm by transesophageal Doppler color flow mapping. Circulation, 74(suppl II):II–132, 1986.

Tamms, M.A., Gussenhoven, W.J., Schippers, L.A., et al.: The value of transesophageal echocardiography for diagnosis of thoracic aorta pathology. Eur. Heart J., 9:1308–1316, 1988.

Theckedath, M., and Nanda, N.C.: Two-dimensional and Doppler echocardiographic evaluation of aortic aneurysm and dissection. Am. J. Cardiol., 54:379–385, 1984.

8

Prosthetic Valves

Surface Doppler echocardiography has become an indispensable tool in the noninvasive evaluation of prosthetic valves. The role of TEE in the evaluation of prosthetic valves can best be appreciated by understanding the strengths and limitations of surface echocardiography. Cross-sectional echocardiographic imaging of a suspected dysfunctional prosthetic valve can identify type and location of prosthesis and presence of thrombus or vegetation as well as give some idea of valve mobility. More importantly, Doppler echocardiographic examination of the suspect valve will give information on the transvalvular pressure gradient, functional valve area, and presence of valvular insufficiency.

Normal Doppler transvalvular velocities vary depending on valve type (in general, higher velocities with porcine and caged ball valves, lower with tilting disc valves) and sewing ring size (smaller ring sizes yield higher velocities for the same type of valve). Transvalvular velocities determined by continuous wave Doppler can be used to calculate transvalvular pressure gradients by the Bernoulli equation:

$$4 \times (V_{max})^2 = \text{peak instantaneous gradient}$$

where V_{max} equals the peak velocity across the valve. Normal ranges for velocities and gradients for individual valves have been published by numerous investigators and recently nicely summarized by Reisner et al.

Because the prosthetic valve transvalvular pressure gradient varies depending on stroke volume (greater flow rates result in higher gradients), significant stenosis may occur with a normal gradient in the presence of left ventricular dysfunction. With Doppler echocardiography, by means of the pressure half-time technique for mitral valves and the continuity equation for aortic valves, accurate prosthetic valve areas independent of cardiac output can be determined. These areas can be compared with established normal areas by Doppler echocardiography to diagnose prosthetic valve stenosis.

Insufficiency of prosthetic *aortic* valves is usually readily diagnosed and accurately semiquantified by surface Doppler echocardiography. Mild aortic insufficiency is present in all mechanical prostheses and should not be considered abnormal. When dysfunction of a *mitral* prosthetic valve, particularly a mechanical prosthesis, is suspected, however, surface Doppler echocardiography may underdiagnose mitral insufficiency because of *masking* of the left atrium by the strong signal of the prosthesis. When clinical suspicion of insufficiency of a mitral prosthesis is high, TEE should be performed.

TEE in Evaluation of Prosthetic Valves

There are at least four situations in which strong consideration should be given to performing TEE in addition to surface echocardiography: (1) suspected insufficiency of mitral prosthesis, especially a mechanical prosthesis; (2) suspected endocarditis; (3) technically difficult surface echocardiogram; and (4) thromboembolic event (Table 8-1).

TEE for Mitral Prostheses

TEE has been clearly shown to be superior to transthoracic echocardiography in assessing patients with mitral prostheses for regurgitation, abscesses, and vegetations. This is primarily due to the location of the TEE probe posterior to and directly contiguous to the left atrium. Ultrasound masking of the left atrium because of the prosthesis hardware is avoided because the left atrium is closer to the transducer than the mitral valve, and the proximity to the left atrium without interposed chest wall structures allows near-field imaging with high-frequency, high-resolution probes.

NORMAL STRUCTURE

Because of the superior imaging capabilities of TEE, each mitral prosthesis can be easily identified and disk or poppet motion assessed. Restriction of opening or limitation in complete closure can be readily determined. Medtronic-Hall valves appear as a single tilting disk with a prominant central strut. The disk opens to 75 degrees and closes flush

TABLE 8-1. Indications for TEE Imaging in
Patients with Prosthetic Valves

Systemic embolic event
Suspected endocarditis
Suspected mitral dysfunction
Technically difficult surface study

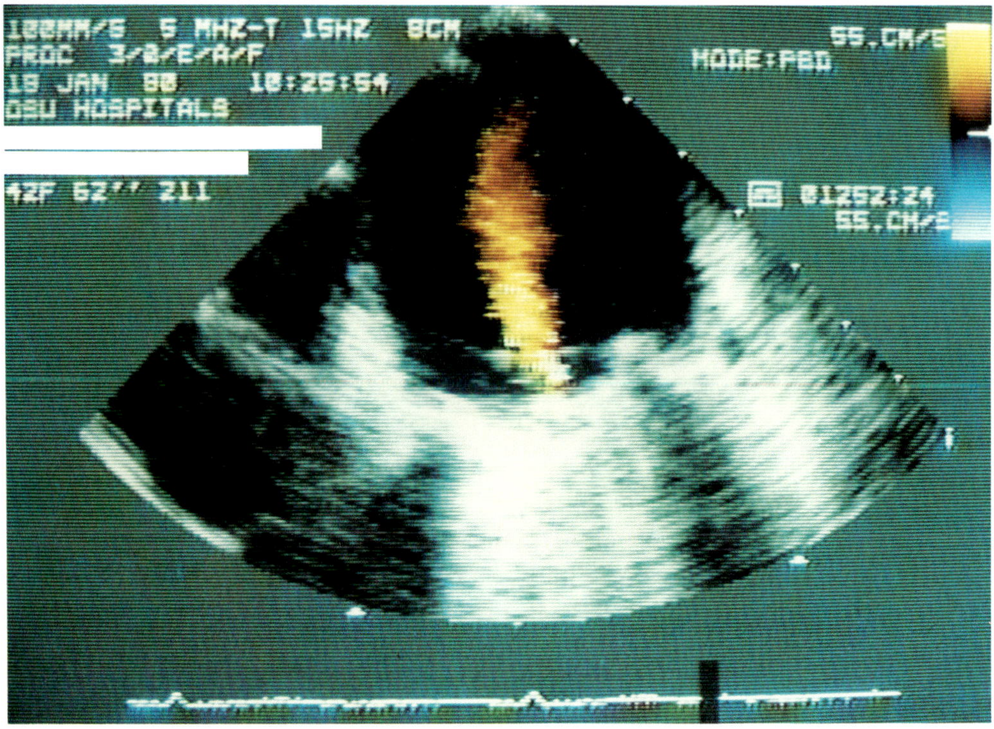

FIGURE 8-1. Normal Medtronic-Hall mitral prosthesis demonstrating prominent central strut and long jet of "physiologic" mitral regurgitation emerging from central hole in tilting disk.

to the sewing ring during normal function (Fig. 8-1). Bjork-Shiley valves have a single tilting disk opening to 60 degrees and also close flush to the sewing ring (Fig. 8-2). In contrast, St. Jude prostheses have two hemidisks opening to 90 degrees and closing at an angle of 45 degrees to the sewing ring (Fig. 8-3). The ball motion with Starr-Edwards prostheses is readily recognized. The ball protrudes approximately 5 mm into the left atrium during systole and moves rapidly and completely out of the atrium during diastole (Fig. 8-4). The normal mitral bioprosthesis when examined by TEE demonstrates thin, mobile leaflets (Fig. 8-5).

MITRAL PROSTHETIC INSUFFICIENCY

The most compelling evidence for the superior sensitivity of TEE is the fact that all tilting disk mitral prostheses demonstrate insufficiency by TEE, whereas only 0 to 38% demonstrate mitral insufficiency by surface echocardiography. Recognition of normal, mild, "physiologic" insufficiency from tilting disk mitral prostheses is crucial in the evaluation of patients with prostheses.

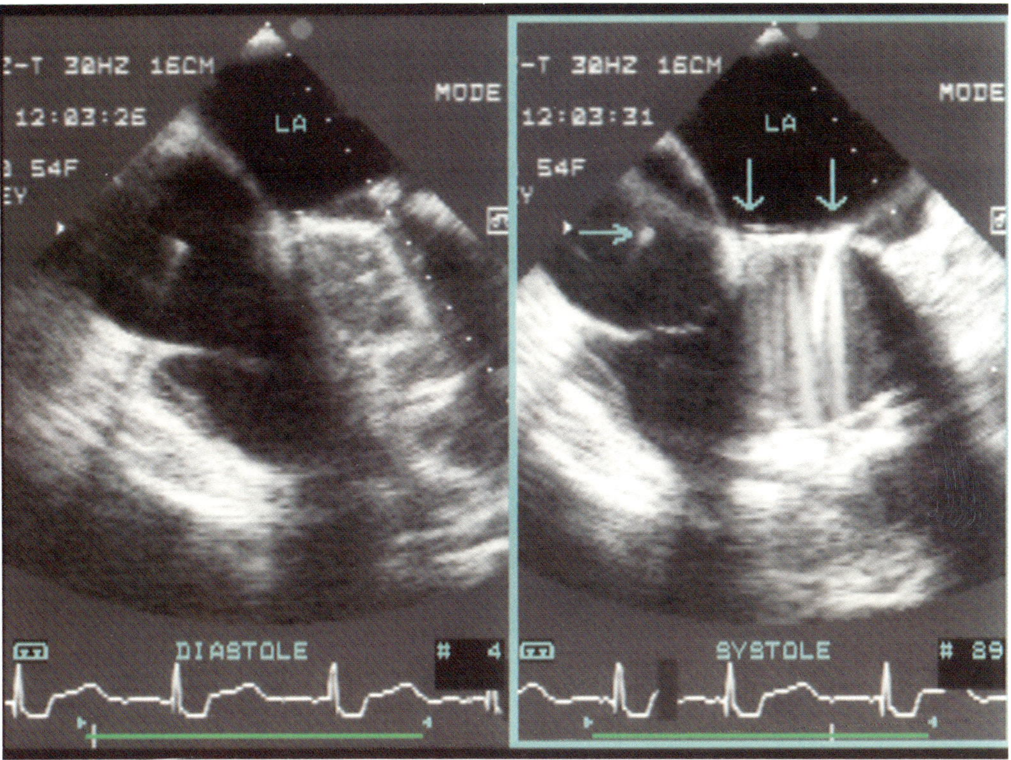

FIGURE 8-2. Normal Bjork-Shiley mitral valve in diastole (left) and systole (right). Horizontal arrow points to pacemaker wire in right atrium. Note closure of disk is perpendicular to sewing ring (*perpendicular arrows on right*).

Taams et al. reported on the color Doppler mitral regurgitant findings obtained by TEE in patients with normal and abnormal Bjork-Shiley mitral prostheses. They described two types of jets: type I, a holosystolic, short (<30 mm), narrow (<10 mm), and predominantly red jet, and type II, a holosystolic, long (>30 mm), broad (>10 mm), or both, and multicolored jet. Type I jets were directed toward the center of the left atrium, whereas type II jets were either directed toward the center or eccentrically directed. TEE Doppler color flow imaging detected two identical type I jets in all 10 patients with clinically normally functioning prostheses. These jets represent regurgitation inherent in the design of the prosthesis owing to (1) blood volume necessary to close the disk and (2) blood volume passing the disk and housing during systole. TEE revealed type II jets in all 10 patients with angiographic or surgical evidence of mitral regurgitation. Seven of these 10 also had type I jets. Interestingly precordial echocardiography detected mitral regurgitation in only six of the 10.

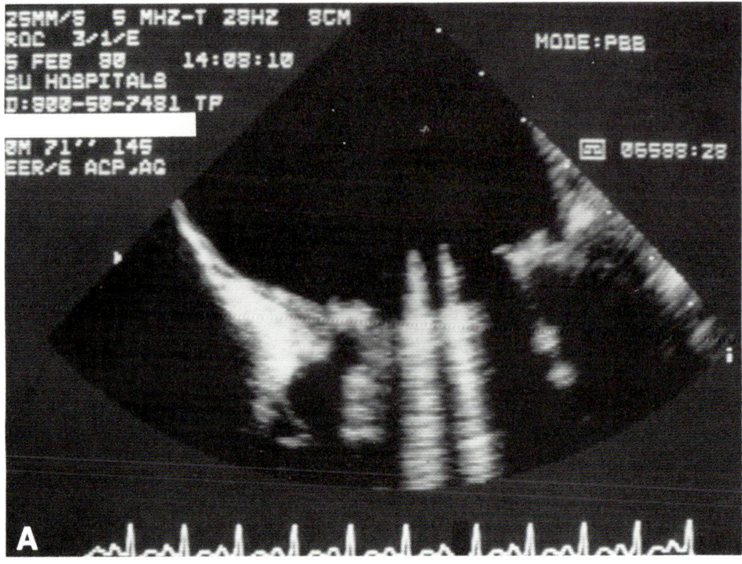

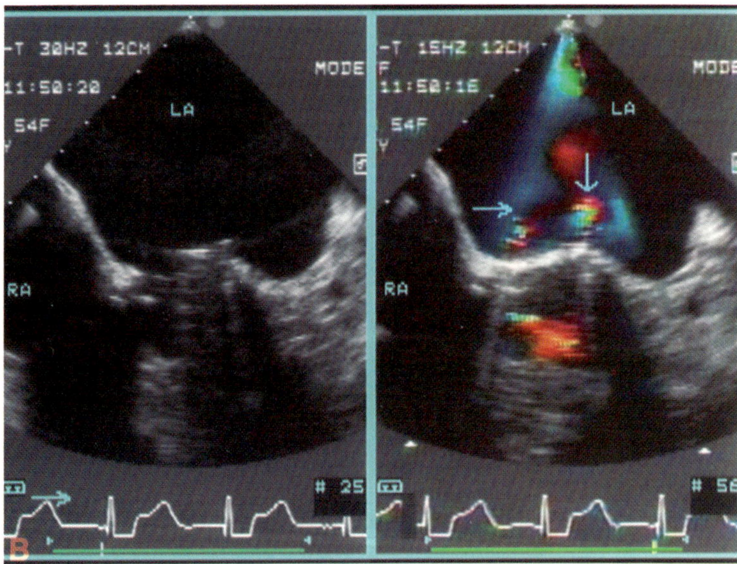

FIGURE 8-3. A. Normal appearance of St. Jude mitral prosthesis in diastole. In this particular patient, orientation of the valve was such that the wide opening of the hemidisks could be appreciated in the transverse plane. B. Systolic frames from normal St. Jude mitral prosthesis. A peripheral and central normal physiologic jet of mitral regurgitation is noted with color flow (*arrows*).

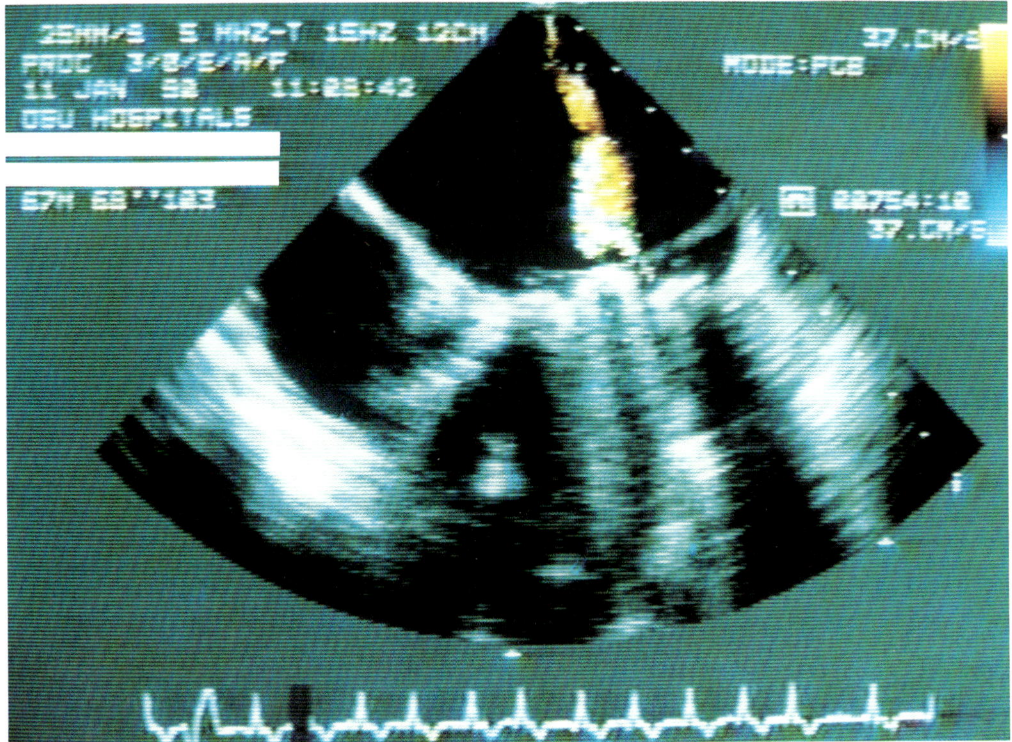

FIGURE 8-4. Holosystolic mitral regurgitation around a Starr-Edwards poppet.

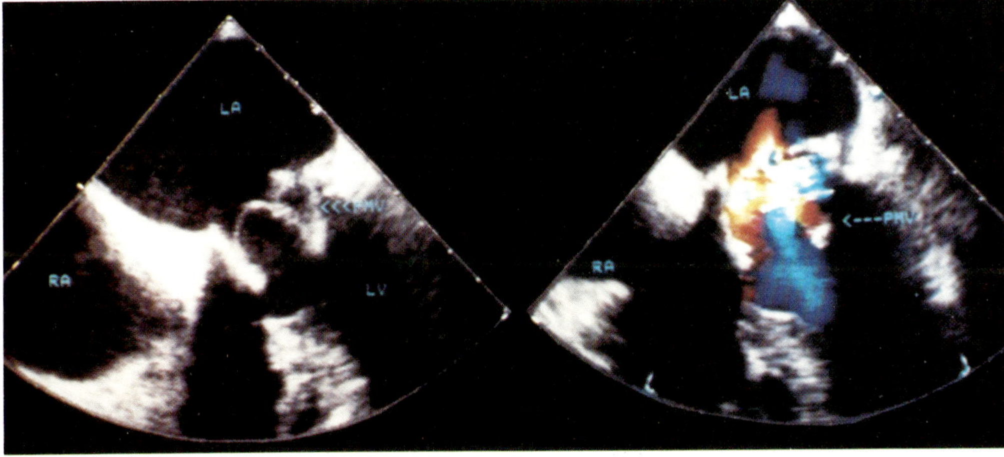

FIGURE 8-5. Normal mitral porcine valve (left). Arrows point to struts. Color flow imaging during systole (right) demonstrates trivial jet of mitral regurgitation.

TABLE 8-2. Characteristics of Normal Regurgitant Jets from Mitral Prostheses

Type of Valve	Jet Location	Jet Length	Timing
Medtronic-Hall	1 Central	3–6 cm	Holosystolic
	2 Peripheral	0.5–2 cm	Holosystolic
St. Jude	1 Central	2–5 cm	Holosystolic
	2 Peripheral	2–4 cm	Holosystolic
Bjork-Shiley	2 Peripheral	2–3 cm	Holosystolic
Starr-Edwards	2 Peripheral	2–3 cm	Early systolic
Bioprostheses	1 Central	0–2 cm	Early systolic

The type and number of mitral regurgitation jets seen by TEE in a normally functioning mitral prosthesis depend on the type of prosthesis. Van den Brink et al. described TEE findings in patients with clinically normal Bjork-Shiley, Medtronic-Hall, St. Jude, and Starr-Edwards prostheses. TEE color Doppler flow imaging demonstrated systolic regurgitant jets originating from the prosthesis in all patients. In contrast, precordial color flow imaging detected none of the regurgitant jets.

Each type of prosthesis generates a specific jet pattern (Table 8-2). Our experience with over 100 mitral prostheses is similar. Bjork-Shiley prostheses exhibit two peripheral type I jets as a result of leakage between the ring and the disk. Medtronic-Hall valves have a very prominent central jet emanating from the center hole in the disk, which can reach lengths of up to 6 cm, and up to two minor peripheral jets (see Fig. 8-1). St. Jude valves demonstrate three small jets of approximately equal size, one central at the central closure line of the two hemidisks and two peripheral between the sewing ring and the disks (see Fig. 8-3).

Our experience with 29 Starr-Edwards prostheses indicates extreme variability in the appearance of mitral regurgitation by TEE for this valve. Approximately three fourths of normally functioning ball and cage valves exhibit either no mitral regurgitation or a very early systolic jet. The remainder, however, may exhibit holosystolic mitral regurgitation jets emerging from between the ball and the sewing ring. Normal recently implanted mitral bioprostheses in our experience demonstrate either no or trivial regurgitant jets with a central origin (Fig. 8-5).

MITRAL PROSTHETIC PATHOLOGY

TEE is now the technique of choice for assessment of mitral prosthetic insufficiency, vegetations, thrombi, and perivalvular abscesses. Several studies have demonstrated the superiority of TEE over surface echocardiography and excellent accuracy in comparison to angiography or pathologic examination.

Nellesen et al. studied 14 patients with clinically suspected mitral prosthesis malfunction by TEE and surface echocardiography. The degree of mitral regurgitation was graded by both approaches according to the size of the jet area and compared with semiquantitative angiographic grading. Measurements were taken in the single systolic frame, where the regurgitant jet reached its maximum extent, and regurgitant severity graded as follows: area <2 cm^2 = mild; area $2–4$ cm^2 = moderate; area >4 cm^2 = severe. TEE assessment of mitral regurgitation agreed with angiographic grading in 13 of 14 cases, whereas surface echocardiography underestimated the severity in eight patients. In addition, TEE provided additional anatomic information not obtained by surface echocardiography in four patients. This included three flail bioprosthetic leaflets and one vegetation. Each of these findings was confirmed at surgery. It should be pointed out that 11 of these 14 prostheses were bioprostheses. In our experience, the additional yield of TEE over surface echocardiography is even greater for mechanical prostheses.

It is not uncommon with mechanical mitral prostheses for surface echocardiography to detect no regurgitation and TEE to detect severe perivalvular regurgitation with subsequent confirmation by angiography, surgery, or both. Examination of mitral prostheses requires meticulous attention to complete interrogation of the entire left atrium from esophageal short-axis to four-chamber views. Not uncommonly, large regurgitant jets caused by perivalvular insufficiency will be di-

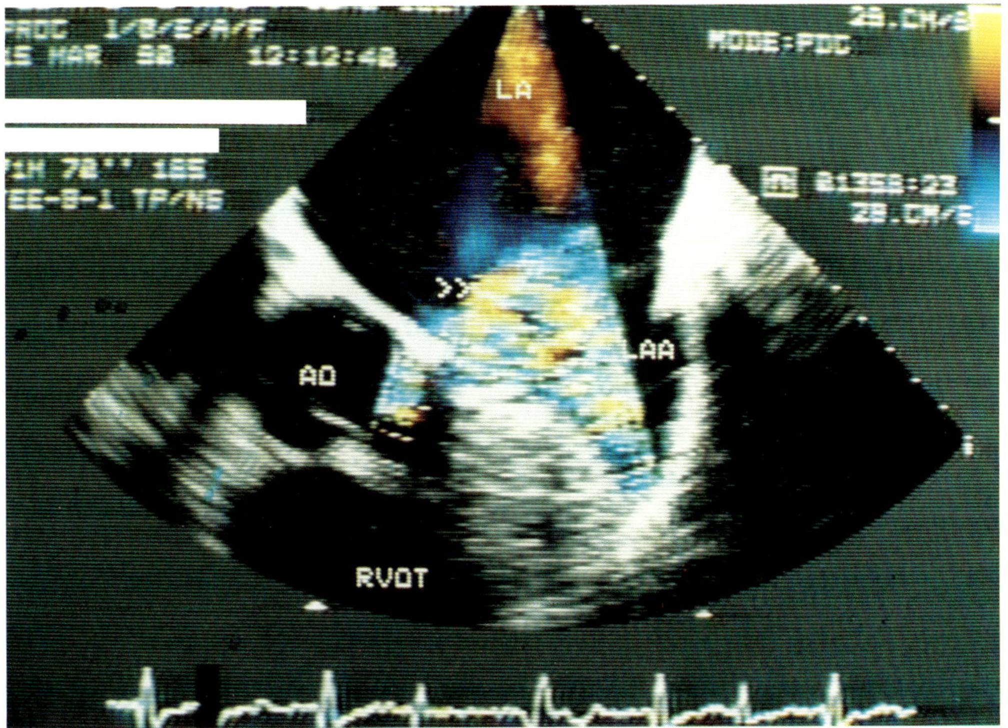

FIGURE 8-6. Perivalvular mitral regurgitation with jet directed into left atrial appendage (LAA).

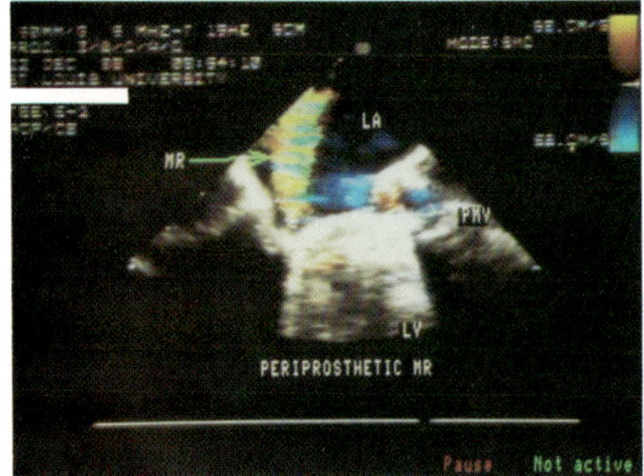

FIGURE 8-7. Medial periprosthetic mitral regurgitation jet.

rected superolaterally into the area of the left atrial appendage (Fig. 8-6). In these cases, marked dilatation of the left atrial appendage can be a clue to the regurgitant jet direction. Medially directed jets in the direction of the atrial septum are usually readily identified from a standard four-chamber view (Fig. 8-7). Large lateral jets as a result of posterolateral dehiscence are also seen well from the four-chamber view

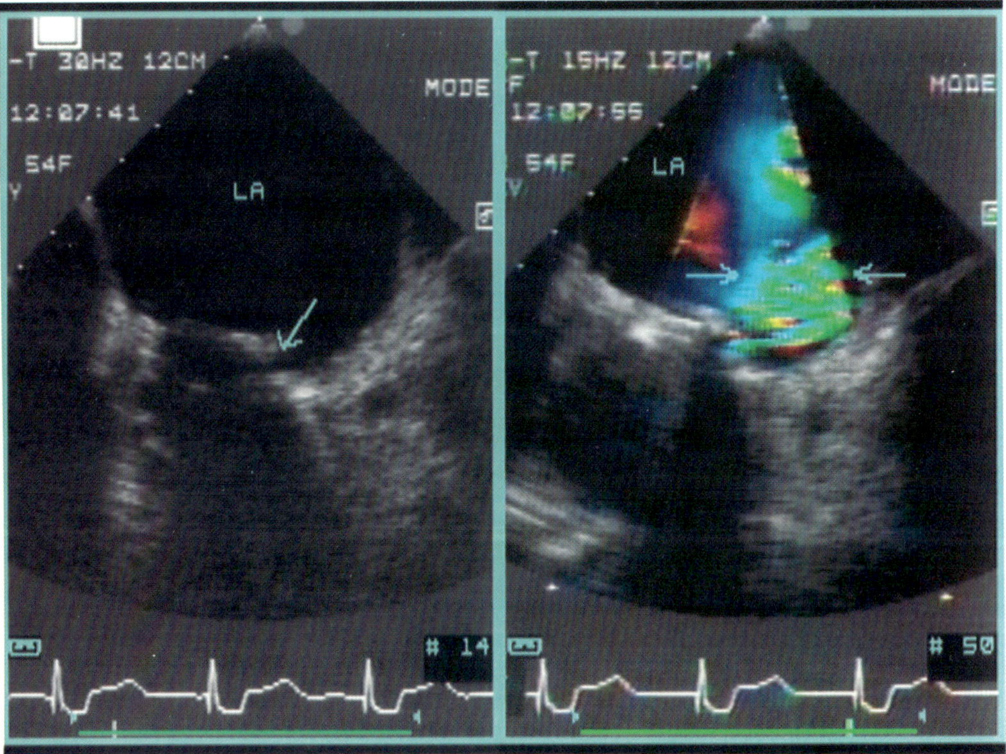

FIGURE 8-8. Lateral dehiscence along with severe perivalvular mitral regurgitation.

(Fig. 8-8). Perivalvular jets as a result of inferior dehiscence that are directed inferomedially or inferolaterally may require nonstandard views, which are between a four-chamber and transgastric short-axis view for imaging.

An important view for assessment of mitral prostheses is the transgastric short-axis view at the level of the valve/sewing ring. In this view, if properly obtained, the entire sewing ring/annulus interface is seen in cross-section, and the site and extent of any perivalvular jets are readily identified (Fig. 8-9). The exact location of dehiscence can be outlined and this information used by the surgeons at the time of re-operation. Degeneration with torn leaflets and mitral regurgitation from bioprostheses are easily recognized from standard views (Fig. 8-10).

TEE is an invaluable tool for the assessment of both native and prosthetic valve endocarditis because of its exquisite sensitivity not only for perivalvular regurgitant but also for vegetations and abscesses. Abscesses appear as echolucent areas between the sewing ring and annulus tissue (Fig. 8-11). Differentiation of a small abscess from normal postoperative charges can sometimes be problematic, and serial studies may be helpful in assessing changes in size.

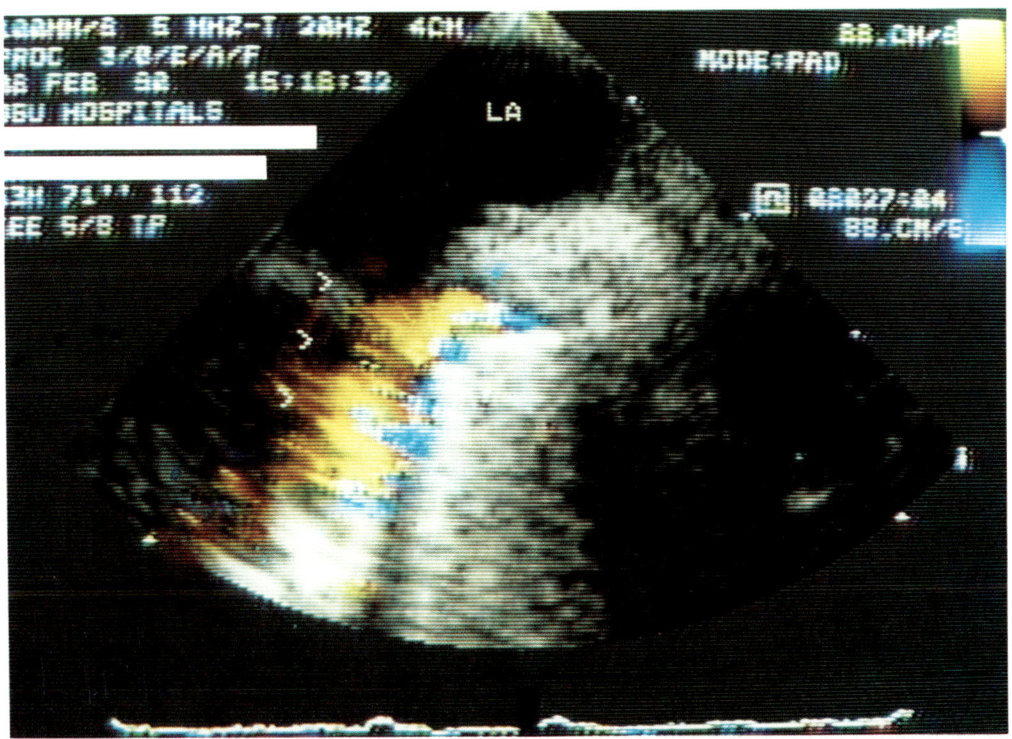

FIGURE 8-9. Transgastric short-axis image at base of dehisced St. Jude mitral prosthesis. A large rim of color emerges on the medial aspect of the sewing ring/mitral annulus interface (*arrowheads*), indicating severe mitral regurgitation.

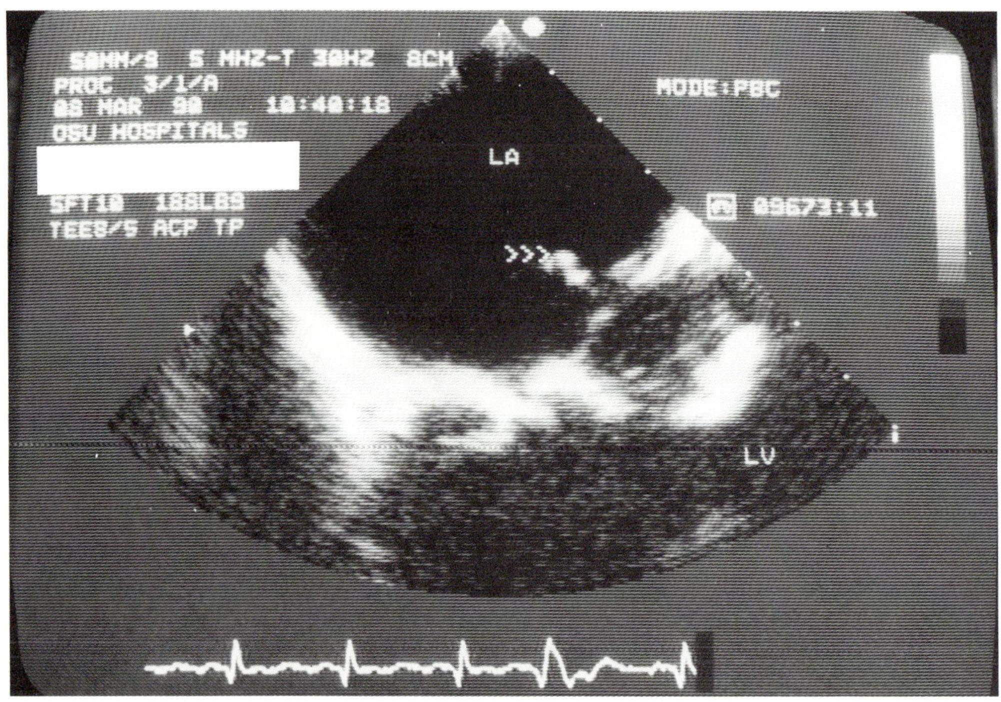

FIGURE 8-10. Torn leaflet (*arrows*) from a degenerated mitral porcine valve.

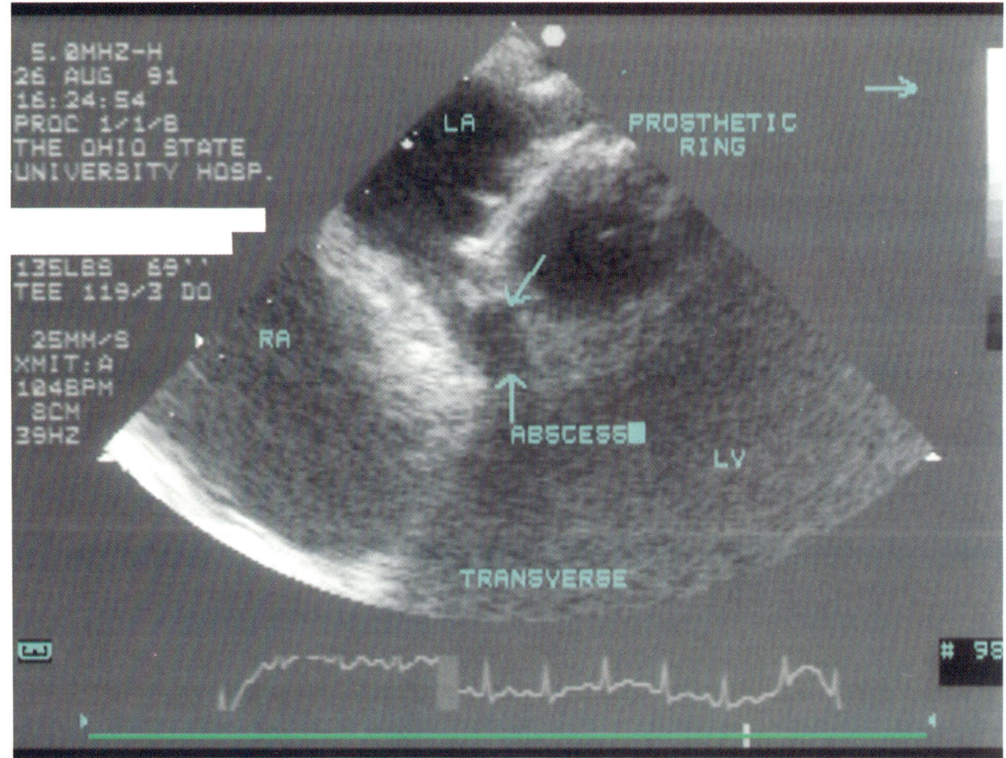

FIGURE 8-11. Transgastric short axis demonstrating septal abscess (*arrows*) at the base of a Medtronic-Hall mitral valve.

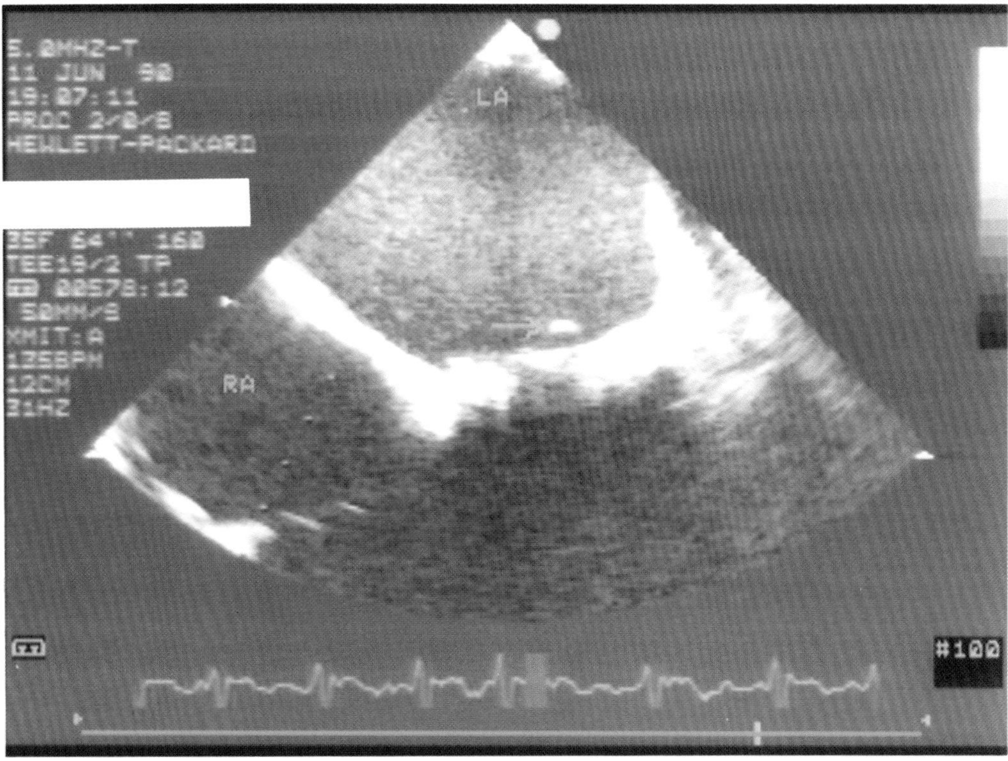

FIGURE 8-12. Small thrombus (*arrow*) on a Starr-Edwards mitral valve in a woman presenting with amaurosis fugax and inadequate anticoagulation.

Detection of thrombus on the prosthetic valve of patients presenting with stroke or transient ischemic attack is greatly enhanced by TEE. We have found surface echo imaging in these situations to be noncontributory. In over 90% of patients presenting with cerebral ischemic events and mechanical mitral prostheses, however, we have found small (2 to 6 mm) mobile strands on the sewing ring of the prosthesis (Fig. 8-12). These structures probably represent small thrombi and have resolved after 4 to 6 weeks of aggressive anticoagulation.

Thrombosis of mitral prostheses is also readily detected by TEE. In these cases, large (1 to 3 cm) pieces of thrombus are detected on the struts of the prothesis with immobilization of the disk (Fig. 8-13).

TEE for Aortic Prosthesis

Many of the situations in which TEE is clearly superior to surface echocardiography with mitral prosthesis apply to patients with aortic prostheses, but certain limitations in the assessment of aortic prostheses must be clearly understood. Both Doppler and two-dimensional interrogation by TEE of the left ventricular outflow tract is somewhat limited

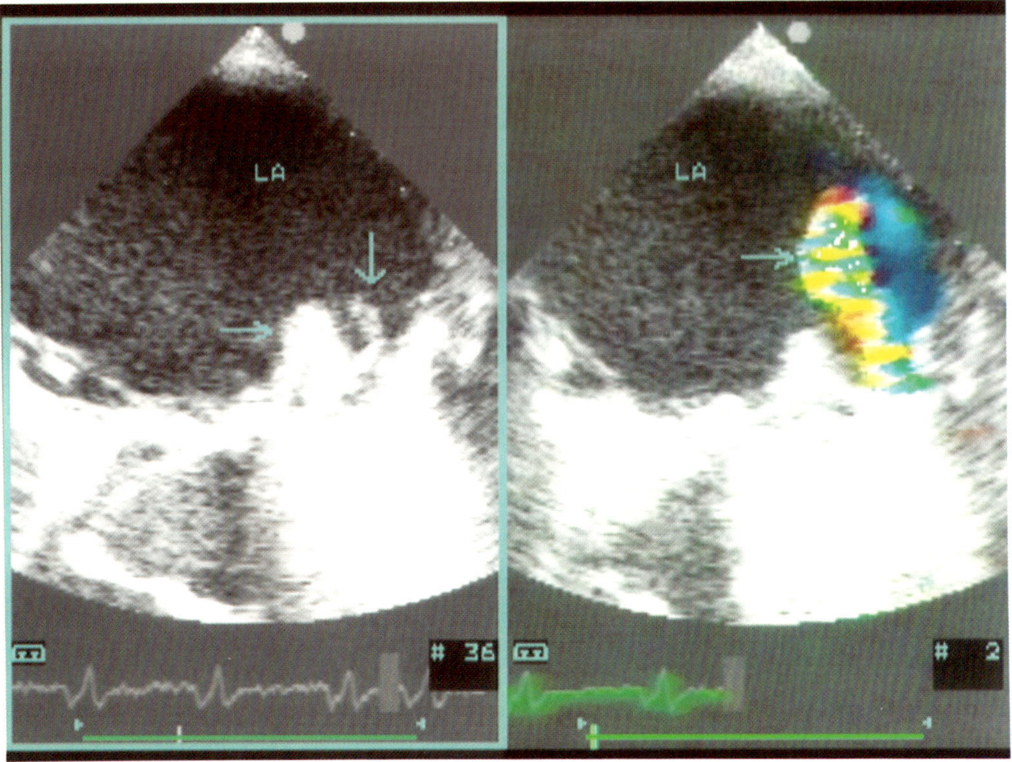

Figure 8-13. Large occluding thrombus (*horizontal arrow*) on the central strut of a Medtronic-Hall mitral valve. A small, more mobile component of the thrombus (*vertical arrow*) is also seen. With color flow imaging, a large jet of mitral regurgitation is noted (*right*).

in the presence of aortic prostheses. The prosthesis itself masks this area because it is usually interposed between the probe and the left ventricle (Fig. 8-14) and flow is not parallel to the transducer. For this reason, assessment of the severity of aortic prosthetic insufficiency may be difficult. In addition, vegetations prolapsing solely into the outflow tract may be missed. Nellesen et al. reported that even with aortic bio-prostheses, the echo signal quality from within the prosthesis was poor and incomplete visualization of the leaflet was noted. No superiority of TEE over surface echocardiography was demonstrated. Fortunately the left ventricular outflow tract is usually well assessed by surface echocardiography parasternal views. Surface echocardiography is also usually very reliable for diagnosing and assessing the severity of prosthetic aortic insufficiency because the outflow tract is unmasked. For these reasons, we recommend a complete evaluation of all aortic protheses by surface echocardiography even if the TEE is believed to be normal. Evaluation of the severity of aortic insufficiency is particularly important by surface echocardiography.

Despite these limitations, TEE can often aid in the diagnosis of aortic prosthetic complications. In particular, the technique should be considered for assessment of anatomic abnormalities, including abscesses and fistulae in patients not responding well to antibiotic therapy (Fig. 8-15). We have found TEE particularly useful in the assessment of patients with suspected endocarditis. For detection of prosthetic aortic root abscess and fistulae, TEE has been invaluable in our experience. TEE findings in root abscess include echolucency around the base of the prosthetic sewing ring with or without perivalvular insufficiency. Differentiation from postoperative changes, especially when aortic graft material has been used, can be challenging. Under these circumstances, serial studies are indicated and will help determine if echolucencies are increasing in size consistent with abscess.

Mohr-Kahaly et al. have reported their experience with TEE in the evaluation of aortic prostheses. Unfortunately comparison with an independent gold standard was not made in this study. In comparison to transthoracic echocardiography, TEE detected transprosthetic aortic insufficiency more commonly (35 of 79, or 44% versus 21 of 73, or

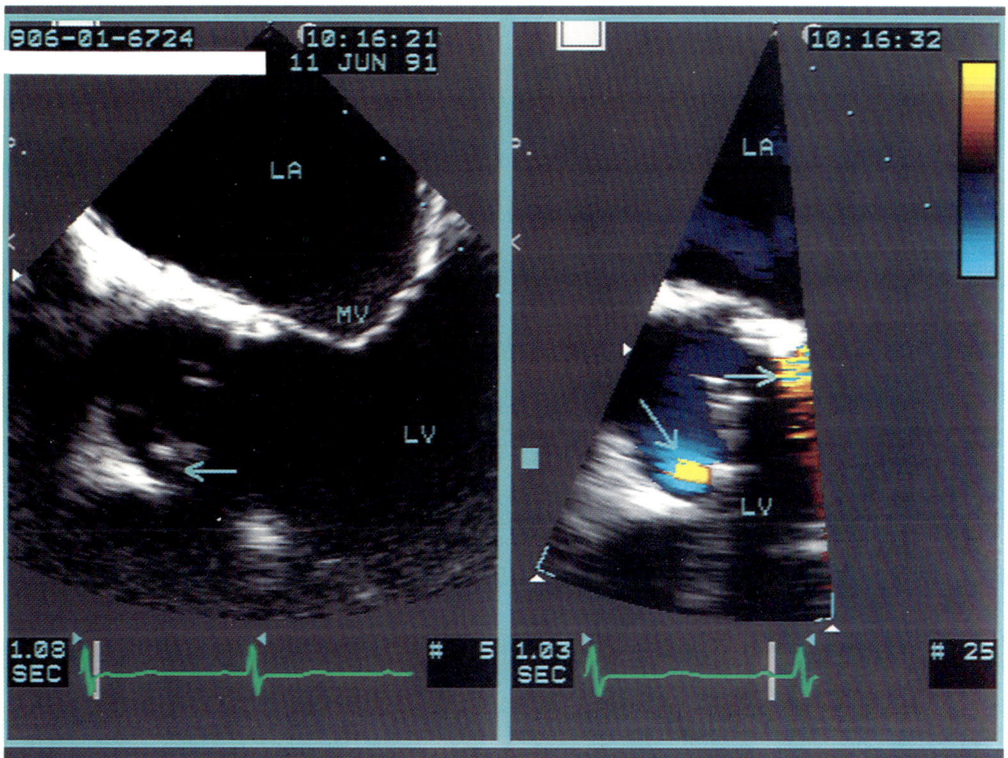

FIGURE 8-14. Prosthetic aortic valve with two perivalvular leaks. Although the outflow tract is partially masked by the sewing ring, the posterior leak can be seen emerging in the outflow tract (*horizontal arrow*). The more anterior leak is suspected by the separation noted with imaging (*horizontal arrow on left*) and the proximal acceleration velocities (*diagonal arrow on right*).

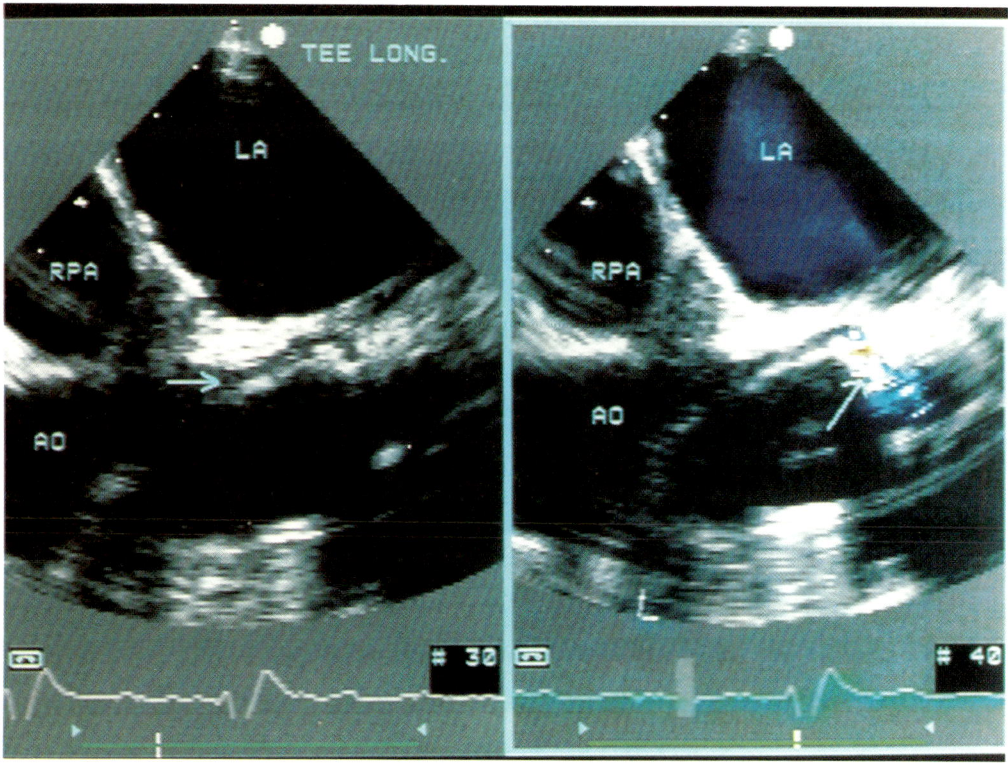

FIGURE 8-15. Longitudinal plane imaging (superior to the left) demonstrating fistulous tract posterior to porcine aortic valve (*horizontal arrow on left*). Color flow imaging demonstrates the perivalvular aortic insufficiency (*diagonal arrow on right*).

29%). In addition, TEE detected complications including vegetations, perivalvular abscesses, and sinus of Valsalva aneurysms with a higher frequency. These investigators believe a regurgitant jet area less than 1 cm^2 and a length of less than 1.5 cm can be considered normal findings for aortic prostheses. This conclusion is supported by in vitro data from Fisher et al., who found aortic regurgitant jets of up to 2 cm in length in normally functioning mechanical prostheses in an aortic flow model.

Bibliography

Alam, M., Serwin, J.B., Rosman, H.S., et al.: Transesophageal color flow Doppler and echocardiographic features of normal and regurgitant St. Jude Medical prostheses in the mitral valve position. Am. J. Cardiol., *10*:871–873, 1990.

Chan, K.L., and Walley, V.M.: Pathologic correlations of transesophageal echocardiographic findings in degenerated bioprosthetic valves (abstract). Circulation, *82(suppl III)*:III–43, 1990.

Cooper, D.M., Stewart, W.J., Schiavone, W.A., et al.: Evaluation of normal prosthetic valve function by Doppler echocardiography. Am. Heart J., 114:576–582, 1987.

Diebold, B., Laperche, T., Raffoul, H., et al.: Efficacy of TEE for making surgical decisions in valvular prosthesis dysfunction (abstract). Circulation, *82(suppl III)*:III–43, 1990.

Dittrich, H.C., McCann, H.A., Walsh, T.P., et al.: Transesophageal echocardiography in the evaluation of prosthetic and native aortic valves. Am. J. Cardiol., *66*:758–761, 1990.

Dittrich, H., Nicod, P., Hoit, B., et al.: Evaluation of Bjork-Shiley prosthetic valves by real-time two-dimensional Doppler echocardiographic flow mapping. Am. Heart J., *115*:133–138, 1988.

Fisher, J.: In vitro evaluation of six mechanical and six bioprosthetic valves. Thorac. Cardiovasc. Surg., *34*:157, 1986.

Nellesen, U., Schnittger, I., Appleton, C.P., et al.: Transesophageal two-dimensional echocardiography and color Doppler flow velocity mapping in the evaluation of cardiac valve prostheses. Circulation, *78*:848, 1988.

Panidis, I.P., Ross, J., and Mintz, G.S.: Normal and abnormal prosthetic valve function as assessed by Doppler echocardiography. J. Am. Coll. Cardiol., *8*:317–326, 1986.

Reisner, S.A., and Meltzer, R.S.: Normal values of prosthetic valve Doppler echocardiographic parameters: A review. J. Am. Soc. Echo., *1*:201–210, 1988.

Scott, P.J., Ettles, D.F., Wharton, G.A., and Williams, G.J.: The value of transesophageal echocardiography in the investigation of acute prosthetic valve dysfunction. Clin. Cardiol., *13*:541–544, 1990.

Taams, M.A., Gussenhoven, E.J., Cahalan, M.K., et al.: Transesophageal Doppler color flow imaging in the detection of native and Bjork-Shiley mitral regurgitation. J. Am. Coll. Cardiol., *13*:95–99, 1989.

Van den Brink, R.B.A., Visser, C.A., Basart, D.C.G., et al.: Comparison of transthoracic and transesophageal color Doppler flow imaging in patients with mechanical prostheses in the mitral valve position. Am. J. Cardiol., *63*:1471–1474.

Williams, G.A., and Labovitz, A.J.: Doppler hemodynamic evaluation of prosthetic (Starr-Edwards and Bjork-Shiley) and bioprosthetic (Hancock and Carpentier-Edwards) cardiac valves. Am. J. Cardiol., *56*:325–332, 1985.

9

Endocarditis

Transthoracic echocardiography has been a valuable technique in the evaluation of patients with suspected infective endocarditis. Demonstration of a vegetation on an affected valve can be helpful in confirming the diagnosis of endocarditis. Furthermore visualization of complications such as abscess formation and hemodynamic abnormalities, most notably insufficiency secondary to infective endocarditis, is invaluable in the management of such patients. Several authors have also reported that the size of such vegetations or even the ability to visualize these lesions by echocardiography offers prognostic information and thereby influences clinical management. Unfortunately transthoracic echocardiography is helpful only in visualizing the vegetation in a subset of these patients. The reported yield of two-dimensional transthoracic echocardiography in patients with infective endocarditis ranges from approximately 50% to 70%.

Role of TEE

TEE appears to be a sensitive technique in demonstrating vegetations on both native and prosthetic valves (Figs. 9-1, 9-2, and 9-3). Studies using TEE indicate that the yield of visualization of vegetations is significantly higher by this technique as a result of the superior resolution and thereby visualization of much smaller vegetations as well as the ability to visualize areas not well seen by conventional transthoracic echocardiography (Table 9-1). Furthermore complications of endocarditis are appreciated with increased sensitivity, including the diagnosis of ruptured leaflets, torn chords, abscess formation, and quantitation of the degree of insufficiency (Figs. 9-4 and 9-5). Daniel et al. reported on a group of 76 patients with infective endocarditis proved by surgery or autopsy. Transthoracic echocardiography revealed vegetations in 60% of the cases. TEE found abnormalities consistent with endocarditis in 94% of these same valves. More impressively, abscess formation was

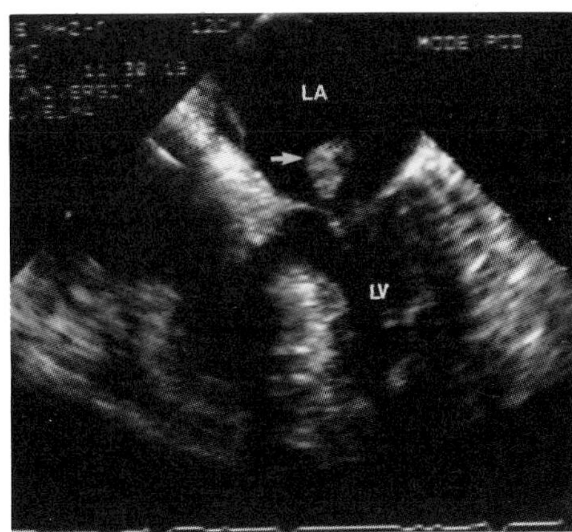

FIGURE 9-1. TEE four-chamber view demonstrating a vegetation (*arrow*) on the mitral valve prolapsing into the left atrium (LA) during systole.

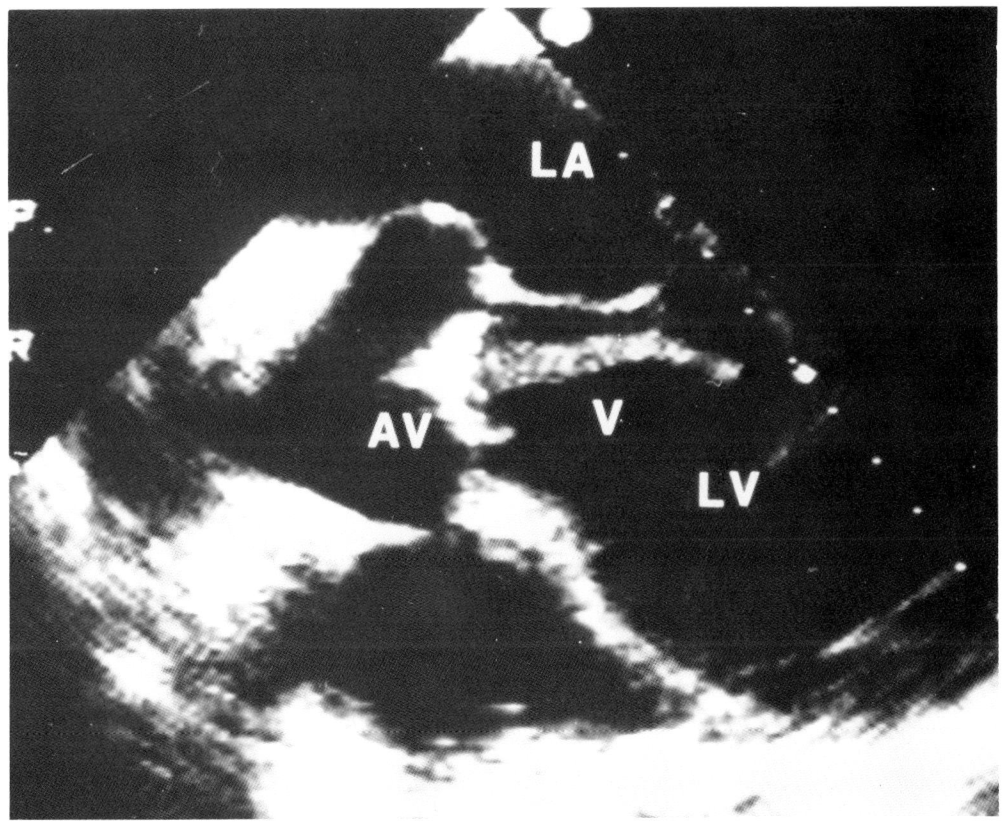

FIGURE 9-2. TEE image showing a serpentine-like vegetation (V) on the aortic valve. This vegetation was not seen by transthoracic echocardiography.

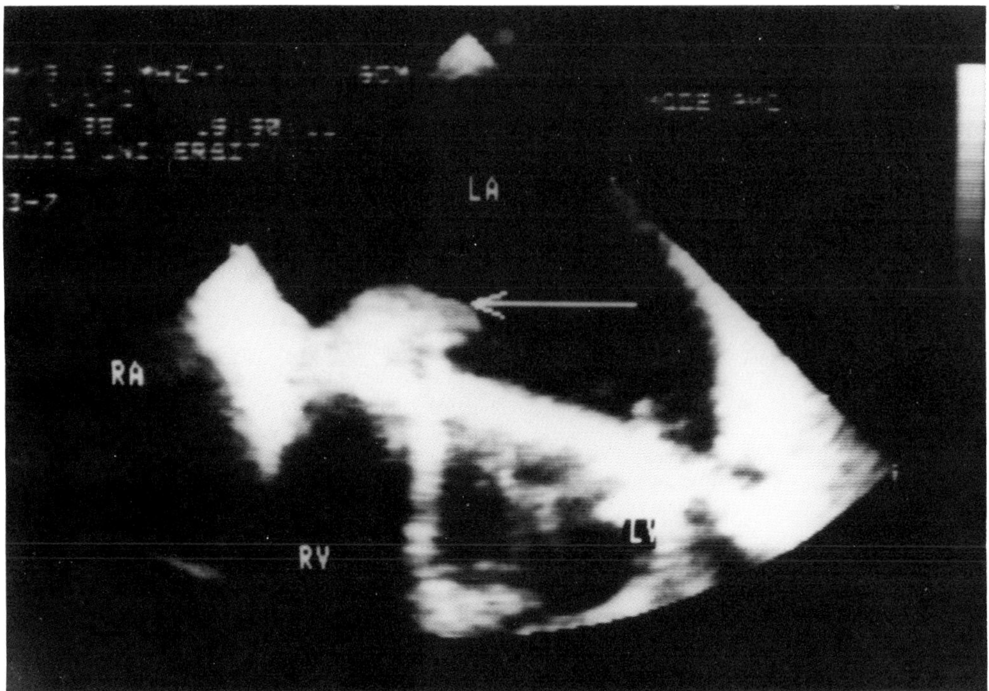

FIGURE 9-3. Infected thrombus (*arrow*) on mechanical mitral prosthesis.

appreciated in 83% of the patients by TEE and only 17% by transthoracic echocardiography. Similarly Erbel et al. reported a much higher sensitivity of TEE in patients with suspected endocarditis. Vegetations were seen in 63% of patients by transthoracic echocardiography and 100% of the patients by TEE. Importantly, only six of 24 vegetations, less than 5 mm, diagnosed by TEE were seen by conventional transthoracic echocardiography (Table 9-2). Mugge et al. reported that the size and mobility of vegetation as seen by TEE identify patients at high risk for subsequent embolic events, particularly with mitral vegetations

TABLE 9-1. Comparison of Transthoracic Echocardiography and TEE in Patients with Endocarditis*

	Sensitivity (%)	
	TEE	TTE
Daniel et al.	97	76
Mügge et al.	96	77
Shively et al.	94	69

* Includes "definite and possible" vegetation.
TTE = Transthoracic echocardiography.

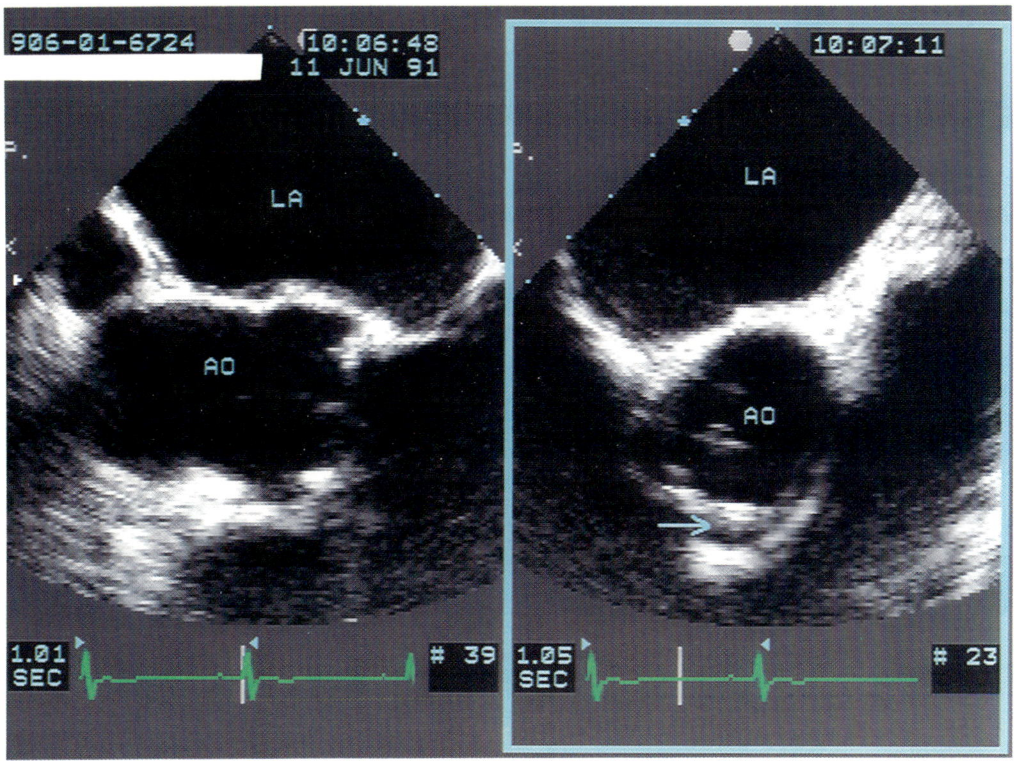

FIGURE 9-4. Horizontal and longitudinal images from a TEE examination in a patient with aortic root abscess formation (*arrow*).

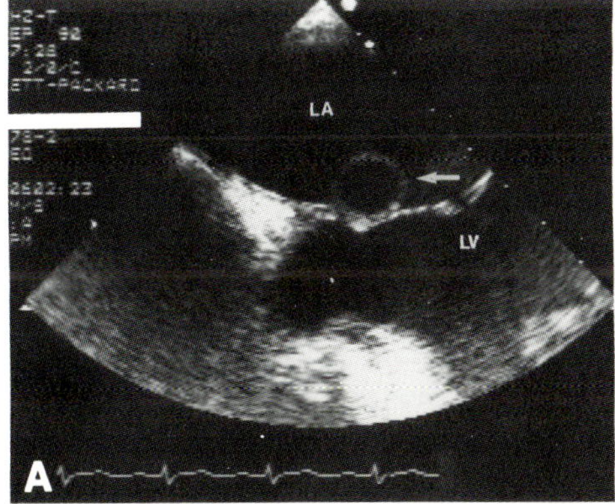

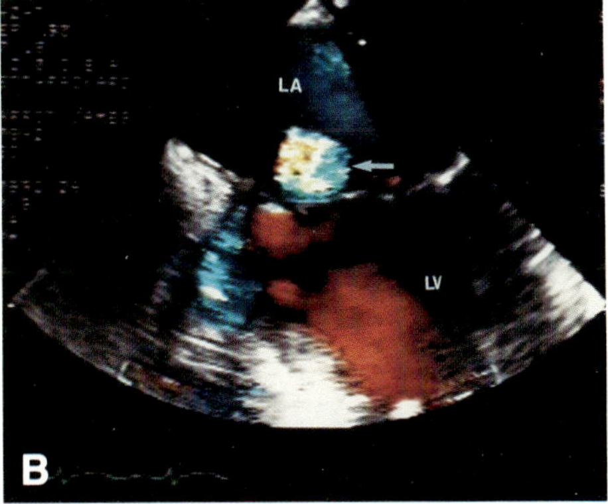

FIGURE 9-5. A and B. Aneurysm of the anterior mitral leaflet secondary to aortic valve vegetation and insufficient jet lesion. (Right) Notice the filling of the aneurysm during ventricular systole (*arrow*).

TABLE 9-2. Relation of Size of Vegetations to Clinical Signs

	Small <5 mm	Medium 6–10 mm	Large >11 mm
TTE	6	9	14
TEE	24	13	14
Positive blood culture	15 (63%)	7 (88%)	12 (86%)
Cardiac murmur	12* (50%)	12* (92%)	13* (93%)
Embolism	4 (17%)	4 (31%)	3 (21%)

* $P < 0.01$, small versus medium, small versus large.
TTE = Transthoracic echocardiography.

From Erbel, R., Rohmann, S., Drexler, M., et al.: Improved diagnostic value of echocardiography in patients with infective endocarditis by transesophageal approach. A prospective study. Eur. Heart J., 9:43–53, 1988.

(Fig. 9-6). These and other studies indicate that TEE is a powerful tool in assessing the patient with suspected valvular endocarditis and in following patients with the diagnosis of the same.

Clinical Application

A great deal of discussion has been generated as to which patients with suspected or known endocarditis should undergo TEE. Arguments can be made for all such patients to have TEE. There are several subsets of patients, however, in whom the procedure is clearly indicated.

Diagnosis

Patients in whom the diagnosis of endocarditis is unclear should undergo TEE. This would include patients with positive blood cultures

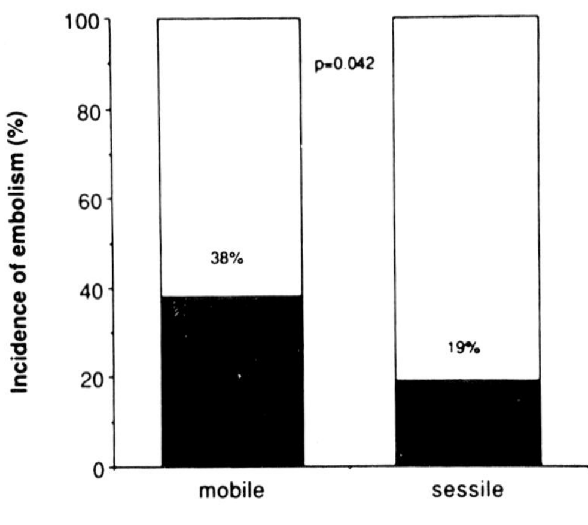

FIGURE 9-6. Incidence of embolic episodes in 68 patients with a *mobile* and 37 with a *sessile* vegetation (black area = embolism). From Mügge, et al.: Echocardiography in infective endocarditis: Reassessment of prognostic implications of vegetation size determined by the transthoracic and the transesophageal approach. J. Am. Coll. Cardiol. *14*:631–638, 1989.

or other stigmata of endocarditis without evidence of endocarditis on transthoracic echocardiographic examination. Although the diagnosis of endocarditis is a clinical one, the finding of a valvular vegetation confirms this diagnosis. The increased yield of TEE in this regard makes it a valuable test.

Prognosis and Treatment

There are several findings on TEE examination that will influence treatment in patients with endocarditis. Although the standard indications for surgery in patients with endocarditis remain (heart failure, persistent infection, and recurrent emboli), findings by TEE may influence the timing of surgery. The finding of severe valvular insufficiency by TEE, for instance, might warrant closer follow-up of an otherwise asymptomatic patient and suggest earlier intervention. Clearly the superior sensitivity of TEE for diagnosing abscess will mean earlier treatment for patients with this complication. Finally, the size and mobility of the vegetation, much better appreciated on TEE, will be a factor in determining optional treatment and timing of surgical intervention.

Bibliography

Daniel, W.G., Mugge, A., Martin, R.P., et al.: Improvement in the diagnosis of abscesses associated with endocarditis by transesophageal echocardiography. N. Engl. J. Med., 324:795–800, 1991.

Daniel, W.G., Schroder, E., Mugge, A., and Lichtlen, P.R.: Transesophageal echocardiography in infective endocarditis. Am. J. Cardiac Imag., 2:78–85, 1988.

Erbel, R., Rohmann, S., Drexler, M., et al.: Improved diagnostic value of echocardiography in patients with infective endocarditis by transesophageal approach. A prospective study. Eur. Heart J., 9:43–53, 1988.

Klodas, E., Edwards, W.D., and Khandheria, B.K.: Use of transesophageal echocardiography for improving detection of valvular vegetations in subacute bacterial endocarditis. J. Am. Soc. Echo., 2:386–389, 1989.

Mügge, A., Daniel, W.G., Frank, G., and Lichtlen, P.R.: Echocardiography in infective endocarditis: Reassessment of prognostic implications of vegetation size determined by the transthoracic and the transesophageal approach. J. Am. Coll. Cardiol., 14:631–638, 1989.

Shively, B.K., Gurule, F.T., Roldan, C.A., et al.: Diagnostic value of transesophageal compared with transthoracic echocardiography in infective endocarditis. J. Am. Coll. Cardiol., 18:391–397, 1991.

10

Cardiac Masses and Cardiac Source of Emboli

Although the vast majority of cerebral infarctions are secondary to cerebrovascular atherosclerotic disease, up to 20% of all strokes are thought to be secondary to cerebral embolism of cardiac origin. Before the advent of TEE, various cardiac imaging modalities yielded disappointing results in demonstrating the cardiac source of these emboli. TEE offers a method for examining regions of the heart often implicated in cerebral embolic events of cardiac origin. These include superior resolution of the left and right atrium and appendages, intra-atrial septum, aorta, patent foramen ovale, atrial septal aneurysm, vegetations, and spontaneous contrast, thus providing increased sensitivity for detection of various cardiac abnormalities associated with cardiac source of emboli. Thrombi and vegetative lesions associated with prosthetic or native cardiac valves are also visualized to a much greater extent with TEE.

Clinical Applications

Evaluation of cardiac source of emboli now represents the most frequent indication for TEE, accounting for approximately 25 to 40% of all studies performed (Fig. 10-1). Identifiable cardiac source of embolus may be divided into abnormalities in which there is definite evidence of cause and effect and lesions that have been found with increased prevalence in patients with cardiac source of embolus of unknown cause (Table 10-1). Figure 10-2 demonstrates the prevalence of various TEE diagnoses in this group. Left atrial thrombus, spontaneous contrast,

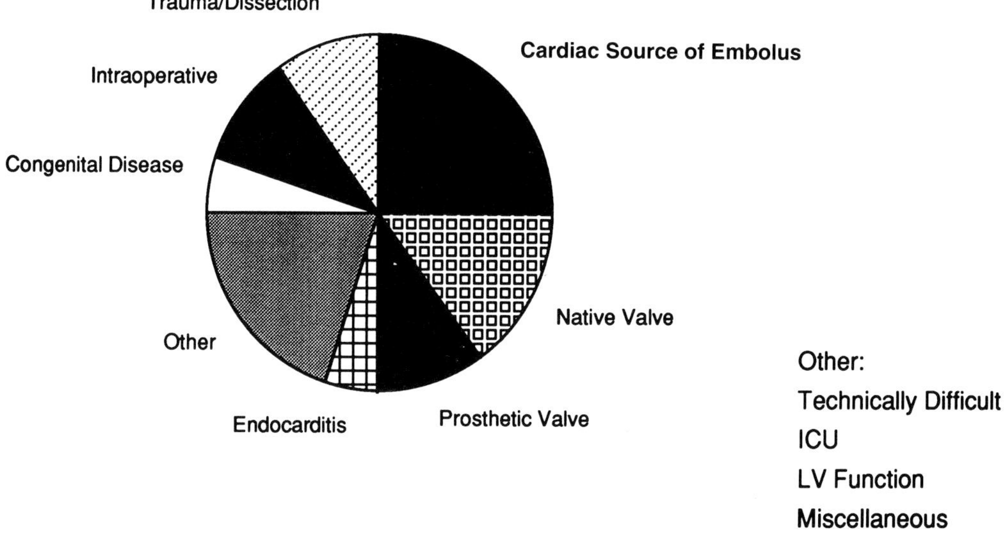

FIGURE 10-1. Percentage of TEE studies performed for various indications. Note that cardiac source of embolus is the largest single indication.

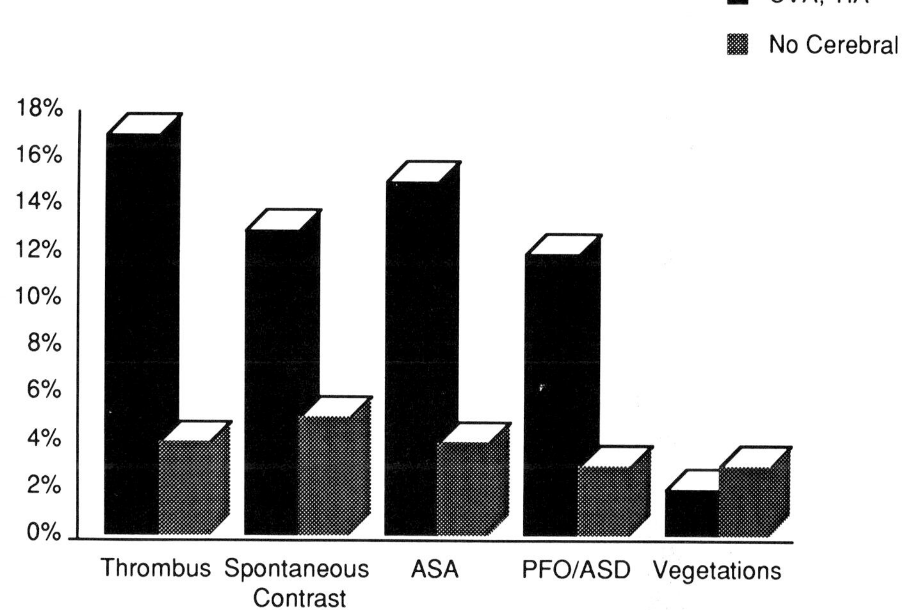

FIGURE 10-2. TEE findings in 250 consecutive patients referred for cardiovascular accident (CVA) or transient ischemic attacks versus 750 patients with no cerebral ischemia. Note the increased prevalence of thrombus, spontaneous atrial contrast, atrial septal aneurysm (ASA), and patent foramen ovale (PFO). (ASD = Atrial septal defect.)

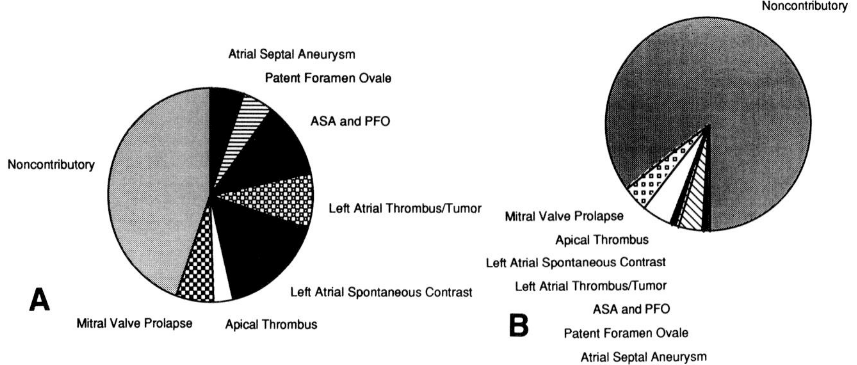

FIGURE 10-3. Comparison of transthoracic echocardiography (A) and TEE (B) in a group of 79 patients with unexplained cerebral ischemia. The yield by TEE was significantly greater.

atrial septal aneurysm, and patent foramen ovale are all seen with greater frequency in patients with unexplained cerebral ischemia than in those without cardioemboli. We have compared the diagnostic yield of TEE and transthoracic echocardiography for cardiac source of emboli in a group of patients presenting with unexplained stroke or transient ischemic attacks. TEE identified potential cardiac source of emboli in approximately 60% of the overall population compared with only 15% by transthoracic echocardiography (Fig. 10-3). Even in patients without clinical heart disease, TEE identified abnormalities in 39% of patients with cerebral ischemic events.

TABLE 10-1. Etiology of Cardiac Source of Embolus by TEE

Definite
    Left atrial thrombus
    Left ventricular thrombus
    Tumor
    Vegetation
    Aortic debris

Probable
    Patent foramen ovale
    Spontaneous echo contrast
    Atrial septal aneurysm

Possible
    Valvular disease
    Wall motion abnormality
    Mitral valve prolapse

Specific Abnormalities

Left Atrial Thrombus

Several studies have demonstrated the superiority of TEE in the identification of left atrial thrombus (Fig. 10-4). The obvious advantage of this technique is the proximity of the left atrium to the transducer location in the esophagus. In standard transthoracic echocardiography, the left atrium is frequently in the far field, in which attenuation of the ultrasound signal hampers identification of such masses. In addition, TEE allows visualization of regions of the left atrium not seen by standard transthoracic echocardiography. This includes, importantly, the left atrial appendage, in which a large number of atrial thrombi can be found. Although it is well known that patients with atrial fibrillation and left atrial enlargement have a higher incidence of left atrial thrombi, several investigators have now shown that left atrial thrombus may be identified in individuals in sinus rhythm with no detectable morphologic or functional cardiac disease (Fig. 10-5). Furthermore decisions regarding anticoagulation of patients, timing of cardioversion, and assessment for percutaneous balloon mitral valvuloplasty are now more comprehensibly assessed with TEE.

Left Ventricular Thrombus

Two-dimensional echocardiography remains the procedure of choice for identification of left ventricular thrombus. The sensitivity and specificity of this technique is in the 80 to 90% range. There is, however, an occasional patient in whom technically adequate transthoracic stud-

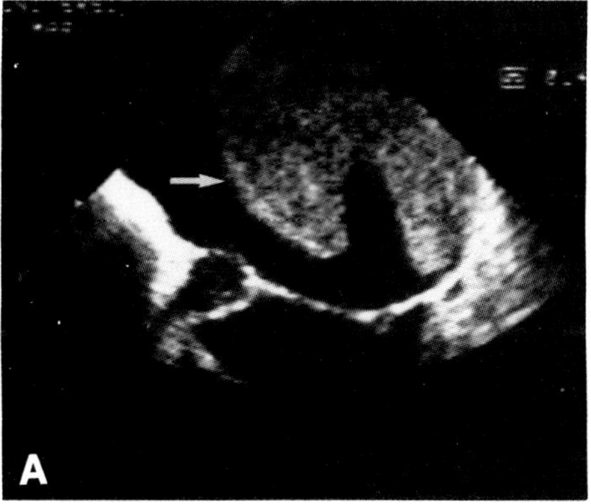
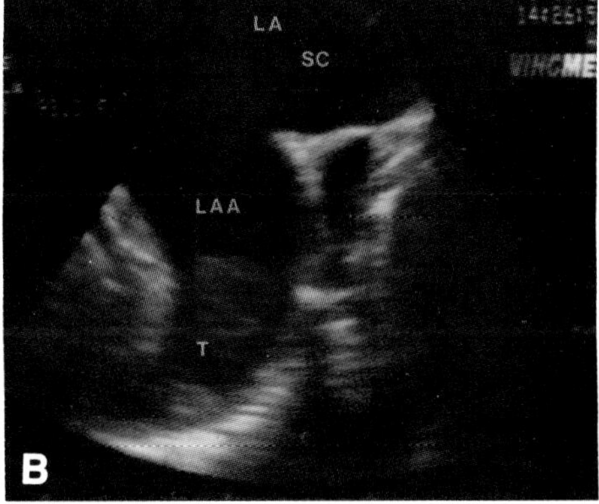

FIGURE 10-4. A. Large left atrial thrombus (*arrow*) in a patient with mild mitral stenosis. B. Thrombus (T) identified in the left atrial appendage (LAA) in a patient with atrial fibrillation. Note the spontaneous contrast (SC) seen in the body of the left atrium (LA).

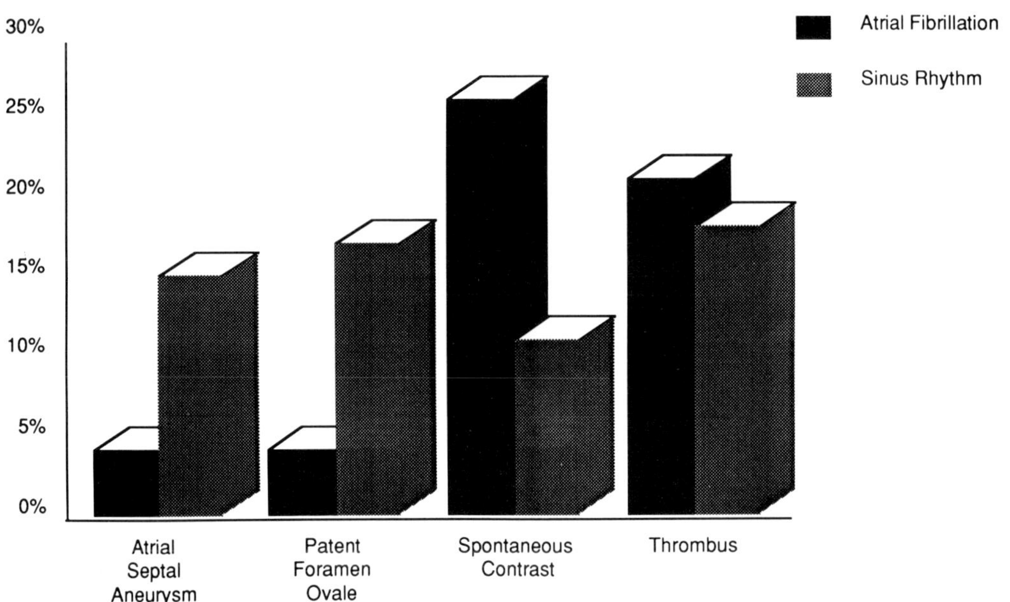

FIGURE 10-5. Abnormalities found on TEE examination in a group of 50 patients with atrial fibrillation and 200 patients in sinus rhythm undergoing TEE examination for identification of potential cardiac source of emboli. Note that the incidence of thrombus is similar between the two groups. Spontaneous echo contrast is found in the left atrium more frequently in the group with atrial fibrillation, whereas atrial septal aneurysm and patent foramen ovale are found more frequently in the group with sinus rhythm.

ies may not be obtainable. In this subset of patients, TEE may be helpful in identifying left ventricular mural thrombus. The operator must be careful to identify the true cardiac apex, which is in the far field of transesophageal images. Visualization of the apex may be enhanced by application of biplane techniques.

Tumor

Myxoma is by far the most common tumor of cardiac origin. These lesions are most commonly encountered in the left atrium, although right atrial myxoma is found in a proportion of these patients. Again, owing to superior visualization of the atria, myxomas are more easily identified by TEE. Identification of the attachment of such lesions as well as differentiation of myxomas from atrial thrombus can best be accomplished by application of this technique. In addition, small recurrent lesions as well as multiple myxomas can be identified with higher accuracy by superior imaging resolutions afforded by TEE (Fig. 10-6). Other tumors that have been associated with cardiac source of embolus include papillomas, fibromas, and carcinomas and have all been identified by TEE in this population of patients.

Vegetations

Vegetations secondary to infective endocarditis are identified with a higher degree of accuracy by TEE (see Chapter 9). It has been shown that the diagnostic yield of two-dimensional echocardiography in identification of vegetations in patients with documented endocarditis is approximately 60%. This yield increases to 90% by application of TEE. More impressive is the yield of TEE in the demonstration of abscess formation in these patients, in whom two-dimensional transthoracic echocardiography is somewhat disappointing. Furthermore characterization of the hemodynamic effects of vegetations can be assessed with a higher degree of accuracy with this technique. Vegetation size and mobility as assessed by TEE are important determinants of embolic potential.

Protruding Aortic Debris

It has been reported that extensive atherosclerotic plaque in the ascending aorta or aortic arch may be responsible for both cerebral and systemic embolization. Protruding and mobile debris appear to have the highest embolic potential. Application of TEE has led to high-res-

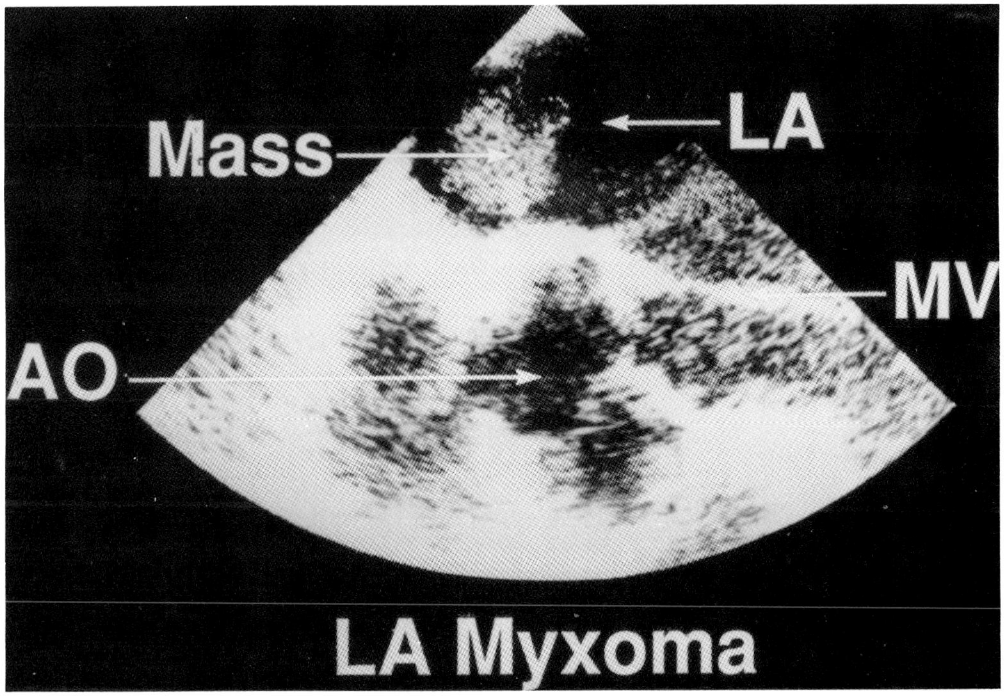

FIGURE 10-6. Basal short-axis TEE view revealing a left atrial myxoma in the upper pole of the left atrium. LA = left atrium; MV = mitral valve; Ao = aorta.

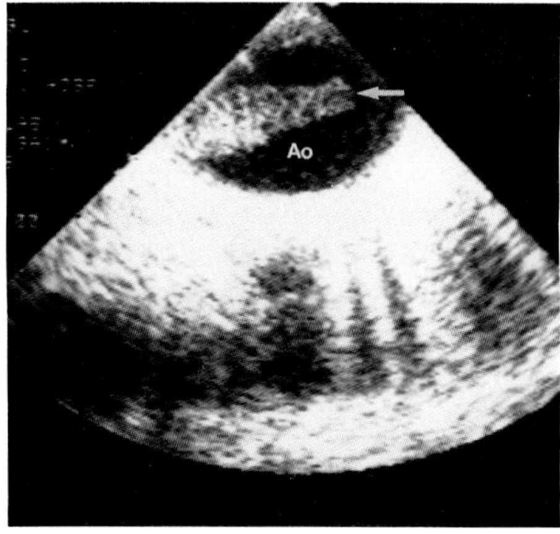

FIGURE 10-7. Protruding mobile debris (*arrow*) in the aortic arch was believed to be responsible for peripheral embolic events in this 55-year-old man.

olution imaging of the aorta. Large protrusive plaques have been identified both in the aortic arch and in the descending aorta in patients with unexplained embolic phenomenon by TEE (Fig. 10-7).

Patent Foramen Ovale and Atrial Septal Defects

Patent foramen ovale and atrial septal defects are known to occur in a significantly higher percentage of patients with cerebral ischemic events than in those with cerebral ischemia (see Fig. 10-2). It has been hypothesized that paradoxical emboli are responsible for the events in such patients. It is clear that TEE is a superior method for the evaluation of intracardiac shunt at the atrial level; with the injection of 10 ml of agitated saline into an arm vein, the sensitivity and specificity of this technique approach 100% (Fig. 10-8). Maneuvers to increase right atrial pressure such as cough or Valsalva may be necessary to demonstrate shunting. Patent foramen ovale is also found in the majority of patients with atrial septal aneurysm and cerebral ischemia (Fig. 10-9).

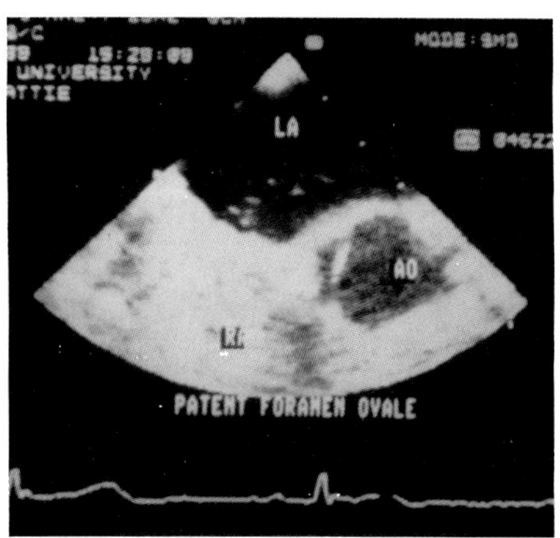

FIGURE 10-8. TEE demonstrating a small patent foramen ovale in a young patient with stroke. Note the passage of agitated saline contrast from right atrium (RA) to left atrium (LA).

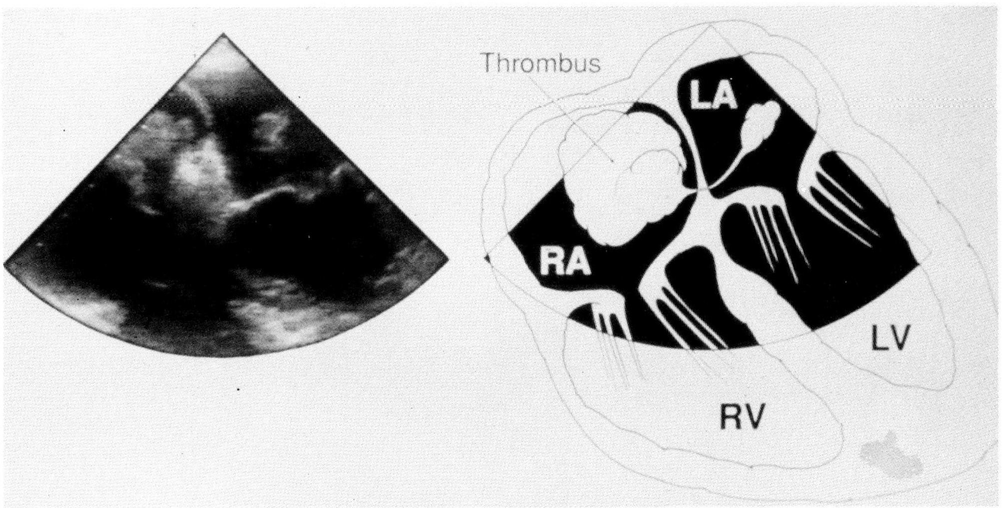

FIGURE 10-9. Demonstration by TEE of a right atrial thrombus extending through a patent foramen ovale into the left atrium. This patient presented with pulmonary emboli and transient ischemic attacks.

Spontaneous Contrast

Spontaneous echo contrast is a demonstration of smokelike swirling reflectances of intracardiac blood flow, most commonly seen in low flow states. Spontaneous contrast is much more commonly seen using TEE than transthoracic echocardiography because of the lack of significant acoustic impedance and the use of higher frequency transducers. The most common clinical setting in which spontaneous echo contrast is found is in patients with enlarged left atria, typically in the presence of atrial fibrillation, mitral stenosis, or both. Spontaneous contrast is also seen in the left ventricle in patients with severe left ventricular dysfunction as well as on the right side of the heart. It has also been described to be present in patients with essentially normal cardiac structure and function when examined by TEE. The finding of spontaneous echo contrast, particularly in the left atrium, has been shown to occur in a much higher prevalence in patients with unexplained cerebral ischemia. Its frequent association with left atrial thrombus suggests that this finding is a marker for blood stasis and subsequent thrombus formation. Studies have demonstrated that this finding in patients with nonvalvular atrial fibrillation identifies a group of patients at high risk for subsequent embolic events (Fig. 10-10).

Atrial Septal Aneurysm

An atrial septal aneurysm is defined as a redundant interatrial septum usually located in the region of the fossa ovalis or sometimes involving the entire interatrial septum, which bulges 15 mm or more

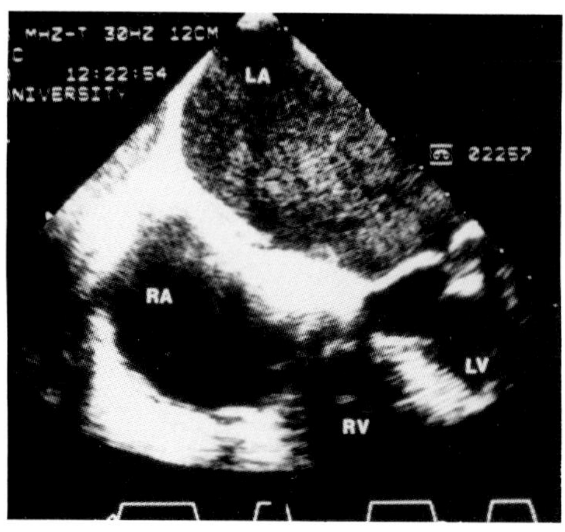

FIGURE 10-10. Demonstration of spontaneous echo contrast in the left atrium in a patient with atrial fibrillation.

beyond the plane of the atrial septum at some time during the cardiac cycle into either the right or the left atrium (Fig. 10-11). This abnormality is reportedly found in only a small percentage of all transthoracic echocardiograms. In the past, however, case reports have identified patients, particularly younger individuals, with cerebral ischemic events and no abnormalities other than atrial septal aneurysms. Using

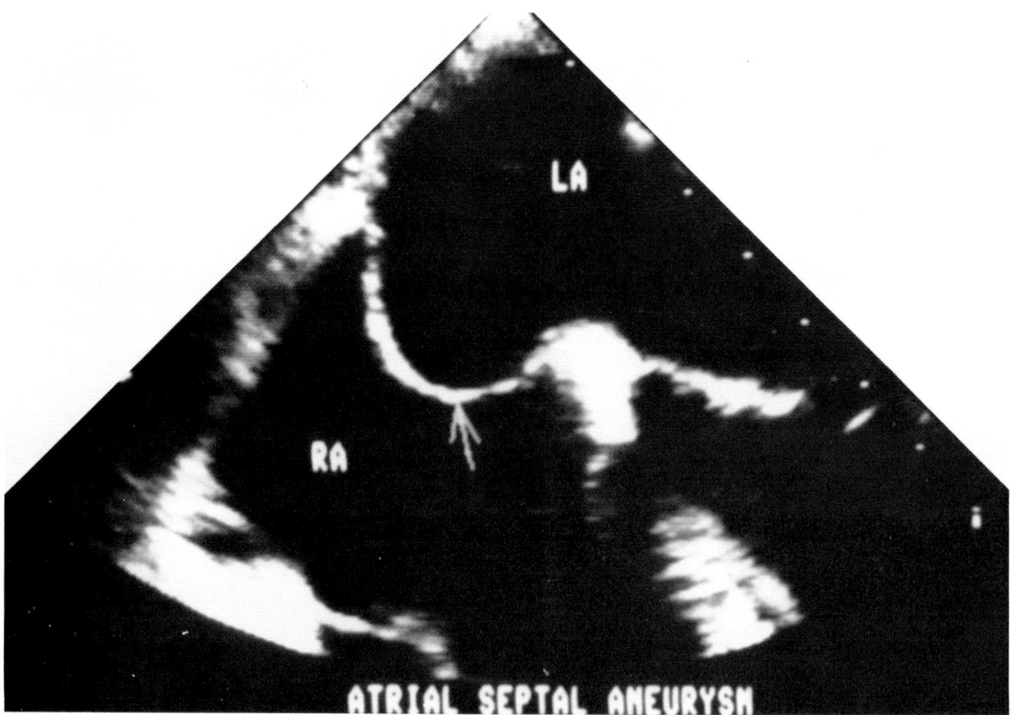

FIGURE 10-11. Atrial septal aneurysm (*arrow*) involving the entire intra-atrial septum and bulging approximately 1.8 cm into the right atrium.

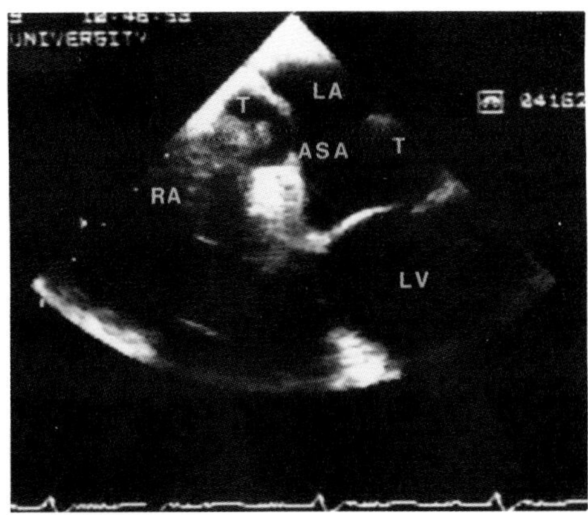

FIGURE 10-12. Atrial septal aneurysm (ASA) with an associated patent foramen ovale in which thrombus (T) can be seen extending from right to left atrium.

TEE, atrial septal aneurysms are identified in approximately 4% of all patients studied. In patients with unexplained cerebral ischemia, however, it may be identified in up to 15% of this population. It has been postulated that perhaps these abnormalities provide a nidus for thrombus formation and blood stasis and therefore constitute a risk factor for cerebral embolization. In patients with unexplained cerebral ischemia, atrial septal aneurysms are associated with atrial septal defects or patent foramen ovale in up to 75% of the cases [and therefore, may be associated with paradoxical emboli (Fig. 10-12).]

Miscellaneous Abnormalities

A variety of other abnormalities have been associated with cardiac source of embolus. These include wall motion abnormalities without documented mural thrombus and isolated valvular lesions including mitral valve prolapse. The diagnosis may also be made more frequently with TEE.

Prognostic and Therapeutic Implications

A recent study revealed the recurrent event rate in those with an abnormal TEE following an embolic event may be as high as 20% at 2 years. Although anticoagulation is certainly indicated in patients with intracardiac thrombus, appropriate treatment in patients with abnormalities such as atrial septal aneurysms and patent foramen ovale remains to be determined.

Bibliography

Castello, R., Pearson, A.C., and Labovitz, A.J.: Prevalence and clinical implications of atrial spontaneous contrast in patients undergoing transesophageal echocardiography. Am. J. Cardiol., 65:1149–1153, 1990.

Black, I.W., Hopkins, A.P., Lee, L.C.L., and Walsh, W.F.: Left atrial spontaneous echo contrast: A clinical and echocardiographic analysis. J. Am. Coll. Cardiol., 18:398–404, 1991.

Kuecherer, H.F., Lee, E., and Schiller, N.B.: Enhanced detection of intracardiac masses by transesophageal echocardiography. Am. J. Cardiac Imag., 4:180–186, 1990.

Mügge, A., Daniel, W.G., Hausmann, D., et al.: Diagnosis of left atrial appendage thrombi by transesophageal echocardiography: Clinical implications and follow-up. Am. J. Cardiac Imag., 4:173–179, 1990.

Pearson, A.C., Labovitz, A.J., Tatineni, S., and Gomez, C.R.: Superiority of transesophageal echocardiography in detecting cardiac source of embolism in patients with cerebral ischemia of uncertain etiology. J. Am. Coll. Cardiol., 17:66–72, 1991.

Pearson, A.C., Nagelhout, D., Camp, A., et al.: Atrial septal aneurysm and stroke: A transesophageal echocardiographic study. J. Am. Coll. Cardiol., 18:1223–1229, 1991.

Schneider, B., Hanrath, P., Vogel, P., and Meinertz, T.: Improved morphologic characterization of atrial septal aneurysm by transesophageal echocardiography: Relation to cerebrovascular events. J. Am. Coll. Cardiol., 16:1000–1009, 1990.

Tunick, P.A., and Kronzon, I.: Protruding atherosclerotic plaque in the aortic arch of patients with systemic embolization: A new finding seen by transesophageal echocardiography. Am. Heart J., 120:658–661, 1990.

11

Congenital Heart Disease

Two-dimensional and Doppler echocardiography have become indispensable tools in the diagnosis and management of pediatric congenital heart disease. The development of these precise noninvasive tools for assessment of cardiac anatomy and hemodynamics has dramatically reduced the need for cardiac catheterization at most pediatric centers. Up to 40% of children in some centers are now referred for operation without cardiac catheterization, with diagnoses made or confirmed by echocardiography.

Babies and young children (under age 5) with unoperated congenital heart disease almost always have excellent ultrasound windows on the heart, allowing complete diagnosis with high-frequency surface echocardiographic probes. Following surgery and with aging, however, these windows become limited and less optimal. In particular, the postoperative congenital heart disease patient may present a challenge for surface echocardiographic examination as a result of the development of fibrous adhesions after midline thoracotomy. In addition, cardiac malformations may be associated with malpositioning of the heart or thoracic or spinal skeletal abnormalities, further complicating the surface echocardiographic examination. Adults with congenital heart disease, either postoperative or nonoperated, are quite commonly encountered in the busy echocardiography laboratory and present a diagnostic challenge. TEE examination plays a significant role in this population.

Even in the adult with technically satisfactory surface studies, TEE examination can provide additional information on structures inherently poorly visualized from the precordial approach. The posterior structures, including pulmonary veins and atrial septum, are almost universally better evaluated by TEE examination. Connections of right atrium to pulmonary artery or right ventricle are much better appreciated by TEE examination than surface echo.

Atrial Septal Defect

Atrial septal defect is one of the most common congenital heart defects in adults. It frequently occurs in isolation. Three main types of atrial septal defect have been described. Most commonly the defect involves the fossa ovalis in the midportion of the atrial septal and is termed an *ostium secundum defect*. In contrast to a patent foramen ovale, the ostium secundum defect involves a true deficiency of tissue. Ostium primum defects are considered a form of atrioventricular septal defect and lie immediately adjacent to the atrioventricular septum, which separates the left ventricle from the right atrium. Atrioventricular canal defects may range from a small ostium primum defect to the complete atrioventricular canal. They are commonly associated with deformity, incompetence, or both of either atrioventricular valve, most often a cleft of the anterior or septal leaflet of the mitral valve.

The third type of atrial septal defect is termed *sinus venosus* and is located high in the atrial septal near the entrance of the superior vena cava. These defects are frequently associated with anomalous pulmonary venous return. Although the sensitivity of two-dimensional echo for the first two types of atrial septal defect is high, the sensitivity for sinus venosus defects is low.

Surface Echo and Atrial Septal Defect

In many centers, two-dimensional echocardiography has replaced cardiac catheterization for the diagnosis of this entity. Direct visualization of the defect in the atrial septum is possible with large defects. Shub et al., using a subxiphoid surface echo approach, found two-dimensional echo sensitive to ostium primum and secundum defects (100 and 89% sensitivity, respectively) but relatively insensitive to sinus venosus defects (44% sensitivity). Color flow Doppler can be used to identify flow characteristics across the defect and may increase diagnostic confidence. With pulsed Doppler, the right heart stroke volume and left heart stroke volume can be calculated and a pulmonic to systemic flow ratio (Q_p/Q_s) estimated.

In our experience, septal dropout is not uncommon even in the absence of a defect. Furthermore blood streaming from the inferior vena cava to the atrial septum can mimic flow across the septum and give the color flow Doppler appearance of an atrial septal defect. For this reason, we perform intravenous agitated saline contrast studies in all patients with suspected atrial septal defect to verify an atrial communication. The appearance of microbubbles, however, in the left atrium either during normal respirations or with a Valsalva may indicate either a patent foramen ovale or an atrial septal defect. We have not found the finding of a negative contrast jet from left to right useful. For these reasons, if contrast studies are positive or the surface study is not optimal, all patients with suspected atrial septal defect at our institutions undergo TEE examination.

TEE in Atrial Septal Defect

A number of studies have clearly established the superiority of transthoracic echocardiographic examination over TEE examination in the assessment of the atrial septum. Hanrath et al. studied 20 patients with ostium secundum atrial septal defects documented at cardiac catheterization by both the TEE and the transthoracic echocardiographic approaches. Two subjects had inadequate surface echocardiograms, and one subject could not tolerate the TEE examination procedure. With the TEE approach, the interatrial septum could be imaged in total in all control subjects as well as in all 19 subjects with atrial septal defect. In all subjects with intact interatrial septum by cardiac catheterization, the interatrial septum was noted rising from the atrioventricular junction to the roof of the atrium. In each of the 19 subjects with a secundum atrial septal defect, a discontinuity of the atrial septum was detected. The size of the defects ranged from 13 to 41 mm. Eleven patients underwent surgical closure of the defects, and the TEE examination estimates of defect size correlated closely with that obtained at surgery. In all 19 patients, contrast shunting from right to left was noted. In contrast, with surface echocardiography the defect could be visualized from the subcostal position in only 10 to 18 subjects (56%). Left-sided echo contrast was seen in only 14 of 18 and negative contrast effect in two of 18 (11%).

TEE examination for atrial septal defect begins by advancing the probe approximately 30 cm from the incisors to the left atrial/aortic level. Slight clockwise rotation should allow visualization of the superior portion of the atrial septum at this level. Slow advancement of the probe will allow scanning of progressively inferior sections of the atrial septum. Ostium secundum defects will be apparent as a discontinuity in the midportion of the atrial septum. Color flow can be superimposed to assess the shunt flow pattern. Figure 11-1 demonstrates characteristic findings by TEE in secundum atrial septal defect.

The size of the defect can be estimated by on-screen measurement of the maximum transverse width (Fig. 11-2). Morimoto et al. studied 11 patients with ostium secundum defect with transesophageal two-dimensional and color flow Doppler echocardiography. Definite visualization of the atrial septal defect was possible in all, and a clear laminar shunt flow could be recorded. The horizontal width of the defects (major axis) was measured from the screen, and the vertical diameter was measured by noting the distance the transducer moved from the rostral to caudal margin of the defect. These defect dimensions corresponded extremely closely to those measured directly at surgery (horizontal width, r = 0.92; vertical length, r = 0.85).

An estimate of the shunt volume can be made by the method of Morimoto et al. Morimoto et al. measured shunt volume across the atrial septal defect directly by placing a pulsed Doppler sample volume in the center of the defect and recording flow. The flow-velocity integral (FVI) can be obtained by planimetry and flow per cardiac cycle calculated as:

$$FVI \times \text{defect cross-sectional area} = \text{shunt flow}$$

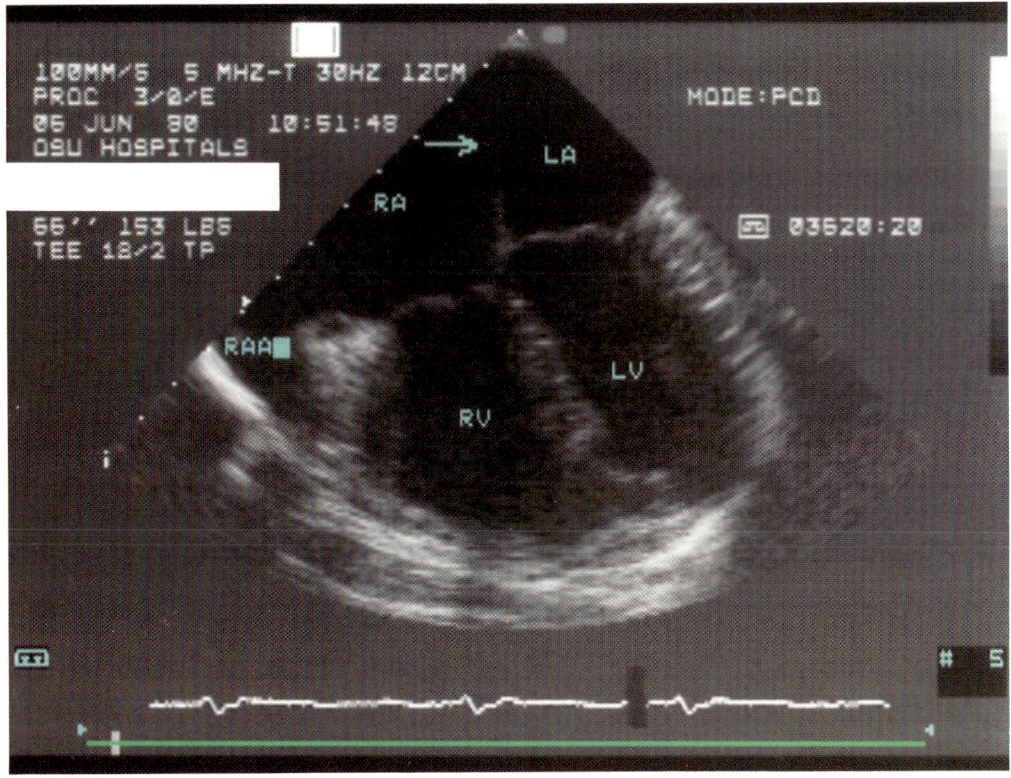

FIGURE 11-1. TEE four-chamber view demonstrating large area of atrial septal dropout (*arrow*). Note the enlarged right atrium, prominent right atrial appendage (RAA), and enlarged right ventricle associated with this large atrial septal defect.

Cross-sectional area is calculated as

$$\text{CSA} = \frac{A \times B}{4} \times 3.14$$

where

A = maximum horizontal width and B = vertical length

To obtain the mean left to right shunt flow velocity during a cardiac cycle, five beats should be averaged (Fig. 11-3). Using this technique, the shunt volume obtained by TEE correlates closely with that obtained at cardiac catheterization using Fick's method.

Larger ostium secundum defects (>5 mm) can be visualized by two-dimensional scanning alone; however, smaller defects may not be seen. Fortunately smaller defects produce characteristic flamelike color flow jets, which are quite prominent and difficult to miss (Fig. 11-4). Very small defects (1 to 3 mm) may be identifiable only by these color flow jets (Fig. 11-4), and the associated defect may be below the limits of two-dimensional resolution. Multiple small fenestrations are not uncommonly seen in patients with atrial septal aneurysm.

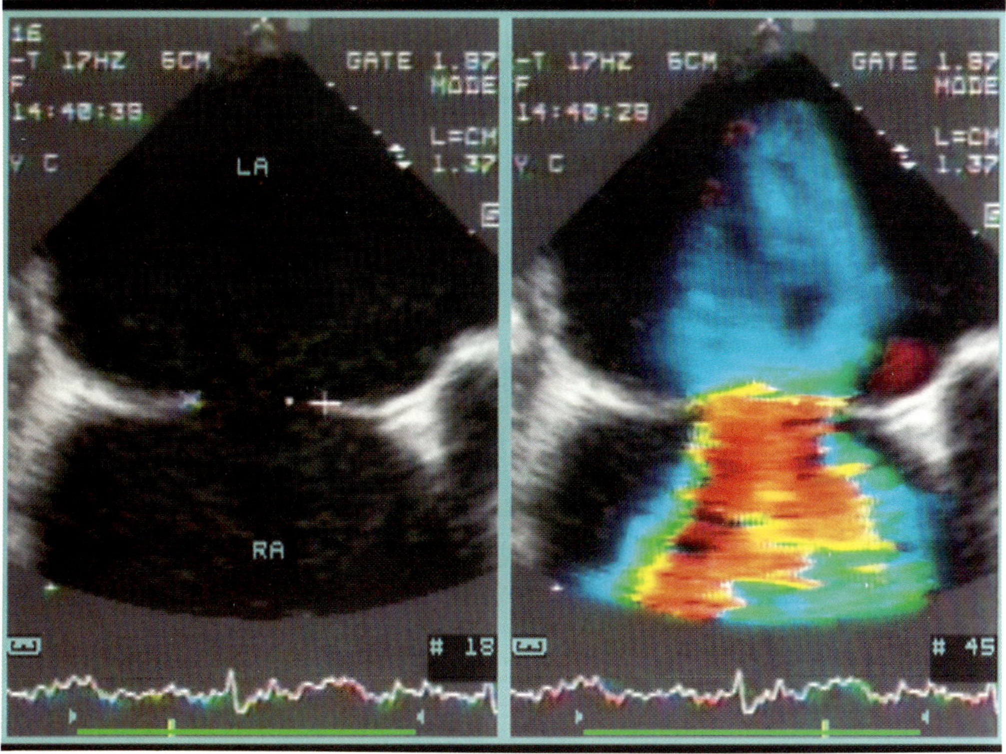

FIGURE 11-2. TEE view of secundum atrial septal defect demonstrating method for measurement of transverse width. With color superimposed (right panel), high velocity, alias flow is seen moving from left atrium (LA) to right atrium (RA). The defect measures 1.37 cm in size. This was confirmed at surgery.

Sinus venosus defects, especially when associated with anomalous pulmonary venous return, may require more meticulous examination for correct diagnosis. A recent study has demonstrated that of eight of 41 atrial septal defects missed by transthoracic echocardiogram, six were sinus venous defects. Careful examination of the superior portion of the atrial septum is necessary. Figures 11-5 and 11-6 demonstrate a sinus venosus defect. Typically the right upper pulmonary vein, which usually passes to the right of the superior vena cava and empties into the left atrium, will be involved with sinus venosus defects. With anomalous right upper pulmonary vein drainage, the vein will empty into the superior vena cava/superior portion of the right atrium at approximately the level of the site of the atrial septal defect (Fig. 11-7). Color flow mapping is extremely helpful in identifying pulmonary vein flow, and the inexperienced transesophageal echocardiographer should spend time during normal examinations identifying all four pulmonary veins and their normal drainage pattern.

The ostium primum defect is easily detected by TEE and appears as a discontinuity in the septum near the crux of the heart.

An exciting new application of TEE reported on by Hellenbrand et

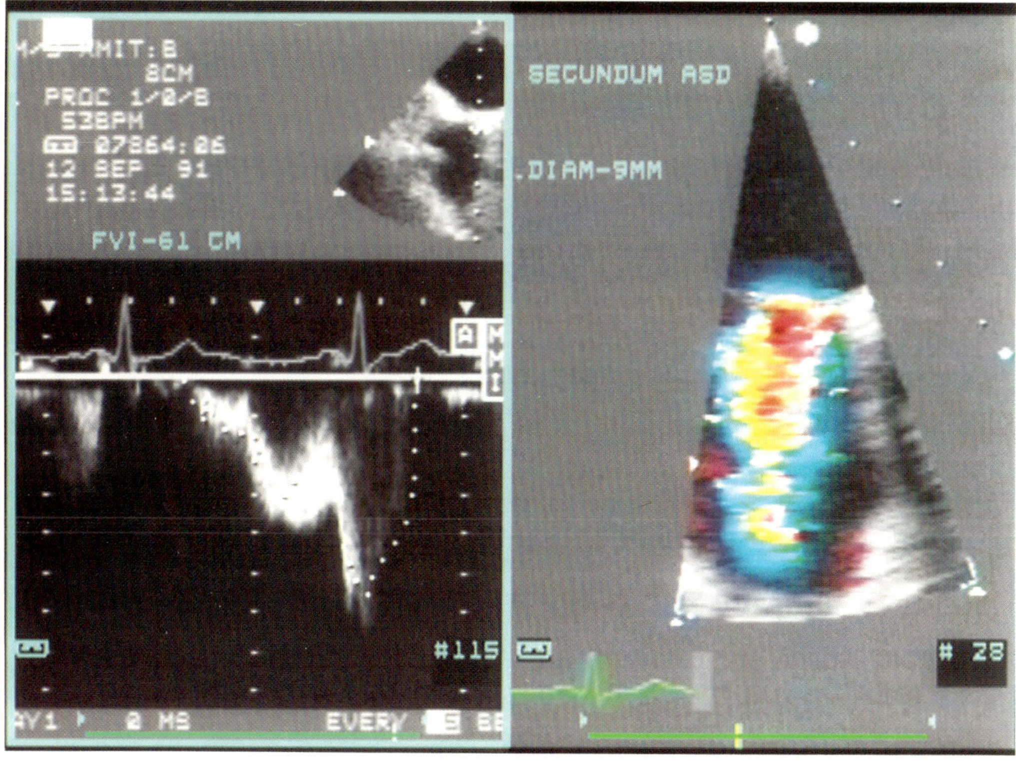

Figure 11-3. Pulsed Doppler recordings (left) of shunt flow at atrial level across a 9-mm secundum atrial septal defect (right). Shunt flow equals 60 cm $\times$ $(^{0.9}\!/_2)^2$ $\times$ 3.14 = 38 ml.

al. is in the transcatheter closure of atrial septal defects. These authors found that concomitant use of TEE with fluoroscopic imaging provided unique and complementary information that improved the efficacy and safety of the technique.

Ventricular Septal Defect

Defects of the ventricular septum are the most common congenital abnormality and occur either in isolation or as part of a complex of cardiac abnormalities. Four major types are usually recognized, with the membranous ventricular septal defect accounting for three fourths. Less common are supracrystal, atrioventricular canal, and muscular defects. The last-mentioned usually are multiple. Ventricular septal defects are frequently associated with additional malformations not recognized as a complex, most commonly obstructive anomalies of the aorta, followed by additional shunts (usually secundum atrial septal defects).

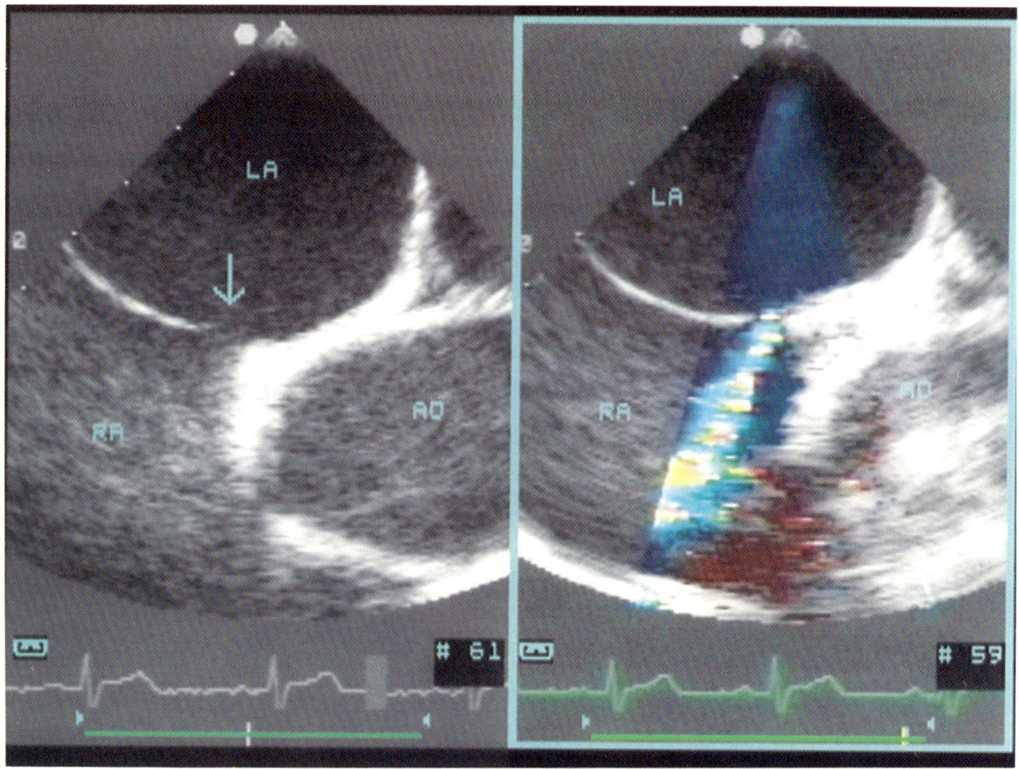

FIGURE 11-4. Longitudinal scan of small atrial septal defect (*arrow*) noted at superior rim of atrial septum. With color flow superimposed (right), a prominent turbulent jet of left to right shunt flow is documented.

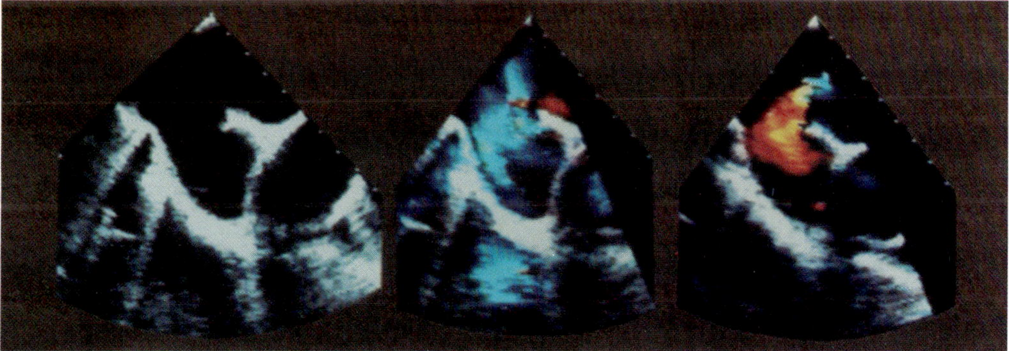

FIGURE 11-5. Large sinus venosus defect visualized in transverse plane (left). Color flow at various times in the cardiac cycle shows left to right (blue in middle panel) and right to left flow (red in right panel) across the defect (*arrow*).

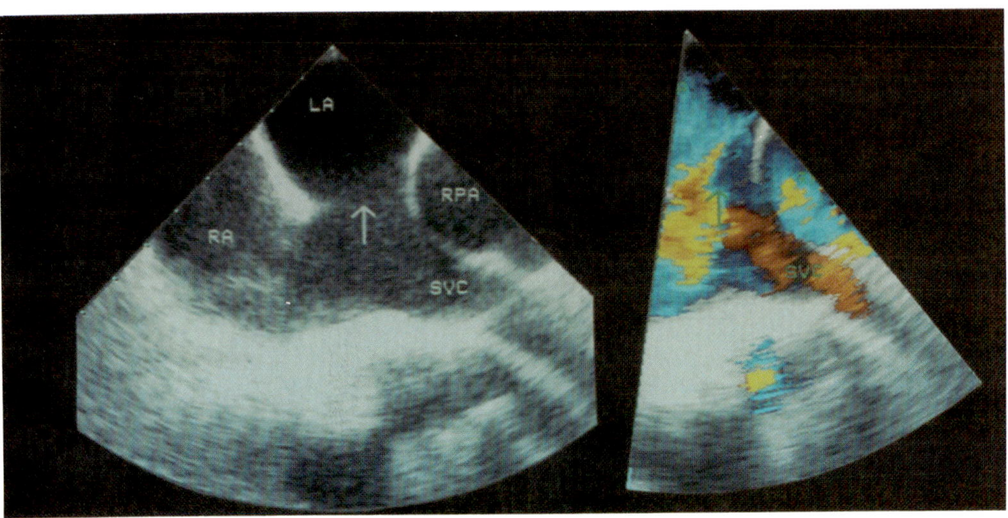

FIGURE 11-6. Longitudinal scan of large sinus venosus atrial septal defect.

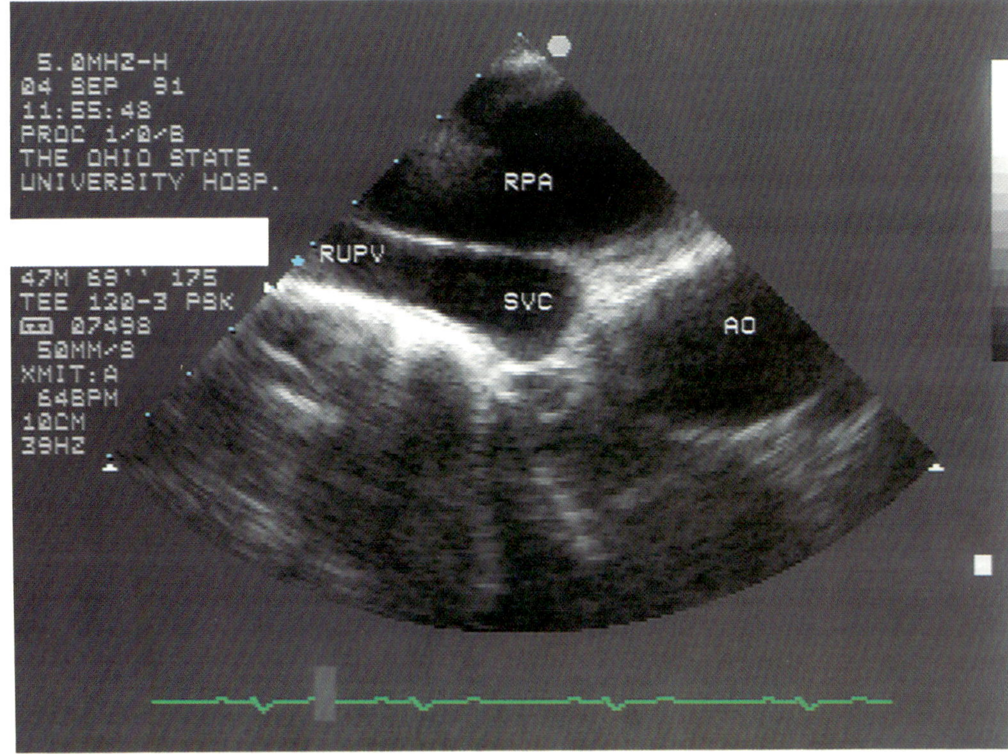

FIGURE 11-7. Transverse plane image of anomalous right upper pulmonary vein (RUPV) draining into superior vena cava (SVC). Note marked dilatation of the right pulmonary artery (RPA).

Surface Echo and Ventricular Septal Defect

Surface echocardiography has proved useful in the detection and quantification of ventricular septal defect. Examination from parasternal long-axis and short-axis windows usually allows direct visualization of medium-sized to larger defects. The addition of color flow Doppler enhances detection of smaller defects, which characteristically generate obvious high velocity and turbulent jets. Continuous wave Doppler can be used to record the velocities across the defect and accurately reflect the right ventricular/left ventricular gradient. As with atrial septal defects, pulmonic to systemic blood flow ratios can be calculated.

TEE in Ventricular Septal Defect

In adults, complete anatomic definition may not be possible with surface echocardiography alone, and TEE is frequently useful, espe-

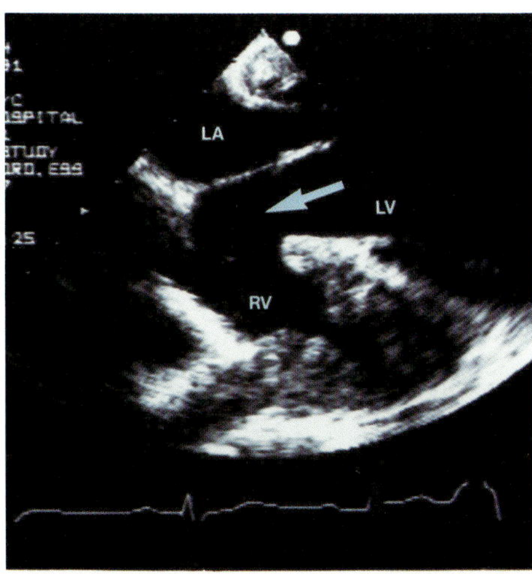

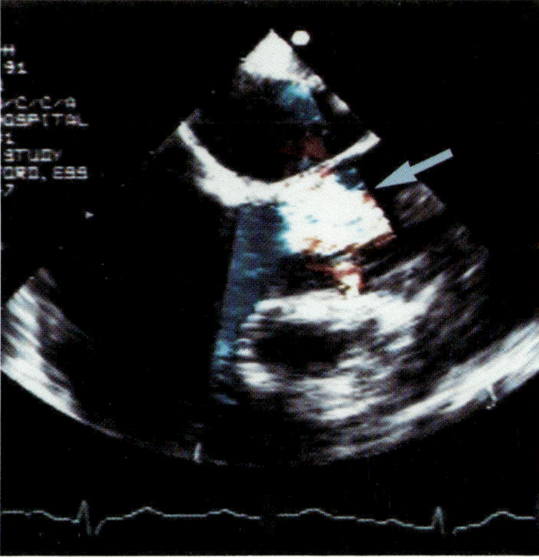

FIGURE 11-8. TEE image of a large membranous ventricular septal defect (*arrow*) with accompanying color flow imaging.

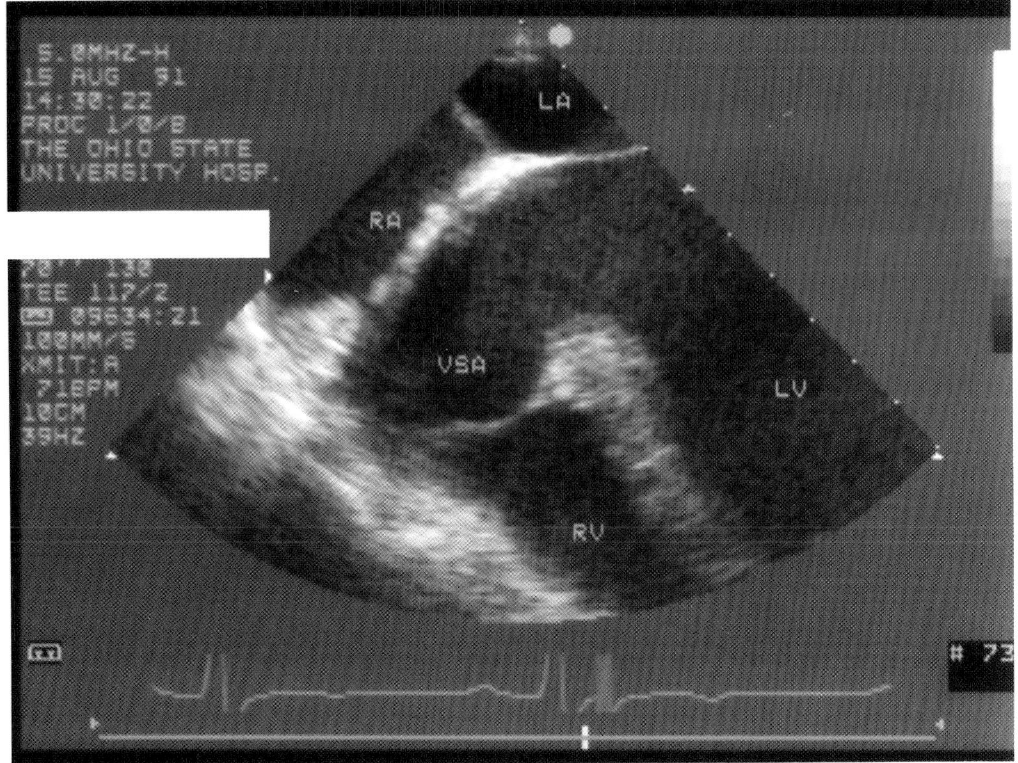

FIGURE 11-9. Large congenital ventricular septal aneurysm (VSA) noted in four-chamber view.

cially in patients with poor precordial windows. Examination for ventricular septal defect by TEE begins with the four-chamber view, with careful attention to the membranous region of the ventricular septum. Figure 11-8 demonstrates a large membranous defect with bi-directional shunting detected by color flow Doppler. Examination in the transgastric short-axis view will also allow visualization of the defect. Small muscular ventricular septal defects are best identified by color flow Doppler either in four-chamber views or transgastric short-axis views. TEE may allow better definition of ventricular septal aneurysms with or without shunt (Fig. 11-9).

Anomalous Venous Connections

Anomalous Pulmonary Venous Return

Entry of all four pulmonary veins into the body of the left atrium can be visualized in the vast majority of patients by TEE. The most common congenital abnormality is anomalous return of the right upper pul-

monary vein in association with sinus venosus atrial septal defect. This
can be identified by careful examination of the area to the right of the
superior vena cava. Normally the right upper pulmonary vein enters
the right atrium at this point. Absence of the vein should suggest anomalous return, and with further examination the anomalous entry more
posteriorly into the left atrium (see Fig. 11-6) is usually easily identified.

Isolated partial anomalous pulmonary venous return can involve different veins and different entry points into the left atrium. In Figure
11-10, a patient with anomalous return of both right pulmonary veins
is presented. At surgery, the entry of the entire right pulmonary circulation into the middle portion of the left atrium was confirmed.

Superior and Inferior Vena Cava

TEE consistently images the entry of the superior and inferior vena
cava into the right atrium. The most common abnormality recognized

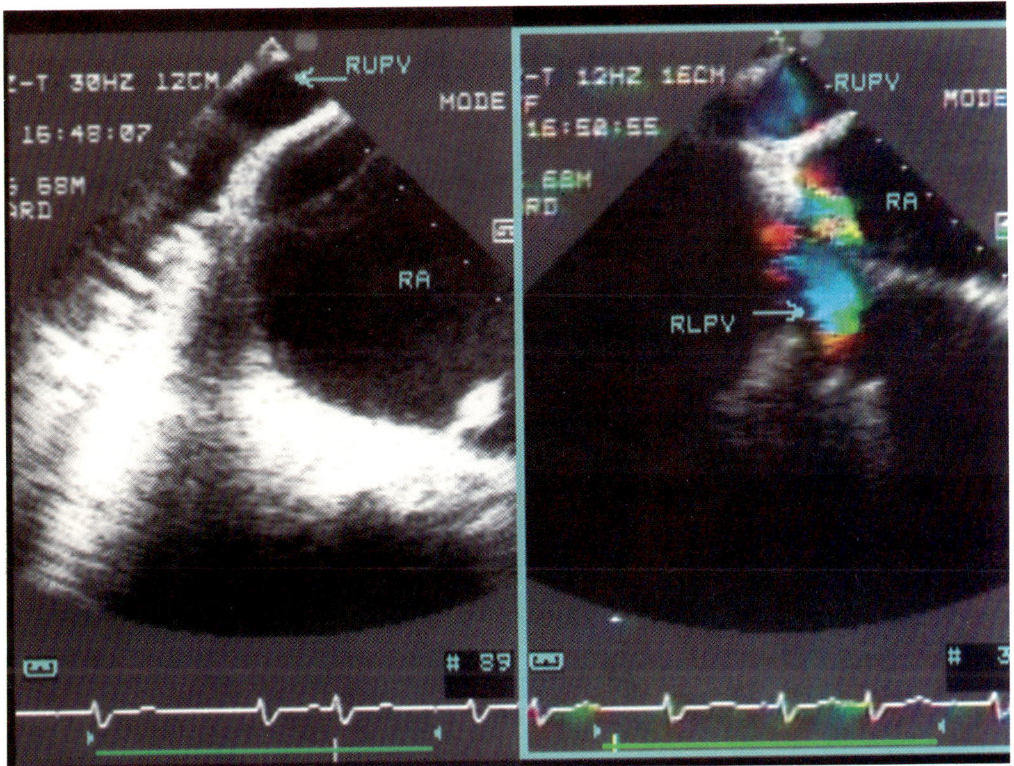

FIGURE 11-10. Anomalous return of both right pulmonary veins. In the left panel, in the upper part of the
esophagus, a large vessel is noted running posterior to the right atrium. This was identified as the right
upper pulmonary vein and emptied into the right atrium at a more superior level. In the right panel, color
flow identifies the right lower pulmonary vein (RLPV) emptying into the lateral inferior portion of the right
atrium. The partial anomalous right pulmonary venous return was confirmed at surgery.

is persistent left superior vena cava. This anomaly can be suspected from surface echocardiographic imaging by the appearance of a markedly dilated coronary sinus. Injection of contrast material into the right upper extremity is followed by opacification of the dilated coronary sinus. With TEE the persistent left superior vena cava appears as an extravascular structure in the sulcus between the left upper pulmonary vein and the left atrial appendage. Slight advancement of the probe or retroflexion allows visualization of the communication between this extravascular structure and a dilated coronary sinus.

Postsurgical Evaluation

Atrial Baffle Procedure

Surgical correction of transposition of the great vessels with an atrial baffle procedure has greatly improved survival in this disorder. Both of the commonly used procedures, however,—the Mustard, which employs a trouser-shaped baffle of pericardium, Dacron, or Teflon, and the Senning, which uses the atrial septum and right atrial free wall for baffle construction—are associated with a significant frequency of late complications. These include nonbaffle complications such as tricuspid regurgitation, right ventricular dysfunction, left ventricular outflow obstruction, and potentially lethal arrhythmias as well as obstruction or leakage from the interatrial baffle.

In young children, surface Doppler echocardiography with examination from the suprasternal, parasternal, and subxiphoid windows has proved extremely useful for evaluation of these baffle complications. In older children and adults, however, the limitation of the precordial window is such that complete evaluation of the systemic and pulmonary venous connections is not always possible. With TEE, complete evaluation of both limbs of the baffle is possible.

TEE examination usually begins with scanning of the liver in a high transgastric position to identify the hepatic vein confluence and the course of the inferior vena cava. The path of the inferior limb of the systemic venous pathway can be traced by slight withdrawal of the probe with counterclockwise rotation. Further withdrawal of the probe allows visualization of the entire systemic venous atrium, the superior limb of the systemic venous pathway, and its anastomosis with the superior vena cava (Fig. 11-11). Identification of the drainage sites of all four pulmonary veins is performed in the usual fashion and the entire pulmonary venous pathway scanned. Obstruction of the superior limb is manifested by narrowing, usually at the junction of the superior limb with the body of the pulmonary venous atrium. Significant dilatation of the superior vena cava usually accompanies this. Interrogation with color flow and pulsed Doppler demonstrates continuous high-velocity turbulent flow at the site of narrowing.

Baffle leaks appear as connections between the limbs of the baffle and the systemic venous atrium accompanied by evidence for blood

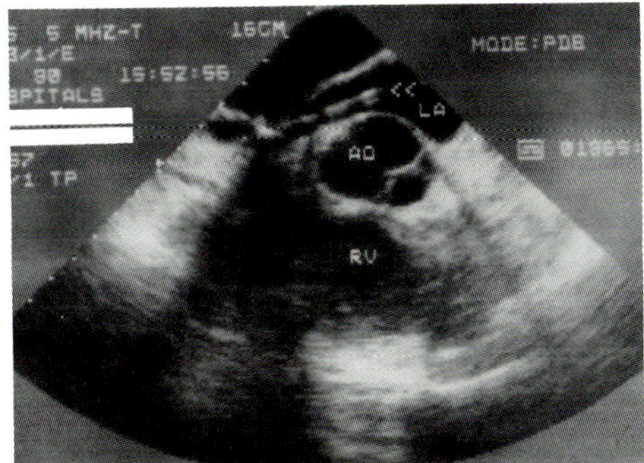

FIGURE 11-11. Visualization of Mustard baffle. A pacemaker wire (*arrowheads*) is noted traveling from the superior vena cava through the superior limb of the baffle and into the anatomic left atrium (venous atrial chamber).

shunting between the two chambers (Fig. 11-12). These occur in both superior and inferior limbs of the baffle and usually at the site of anastomosis.

TEE appears to be the method of choice for assessment of atrial baffles. Kaulitz et al. studied 15 patients aged 3 to 33 years who had undergone Mustard or Senning procedures with both TEE and transthoracic echocardiography. The transthoracic echocardiogram, although able to visualize the supramitral portion of the common systemic venous atrium in every case, identified superior limb obstruction in only three of six patients, midbaffle obstruction in zero of two, and inferior limb obstruction in zero of two. The pulmonary venous atrium was equally well interrogated by TEE and transthoracic echocardiography, with both techniques identifying three cases of midpulmonary venous atrium obstruction; however, only TEE was able to record individual pulmonary vein velocity profiles. Baffle leaks were identified by TEE in 11 cases, only three of which were identified by surface echo.

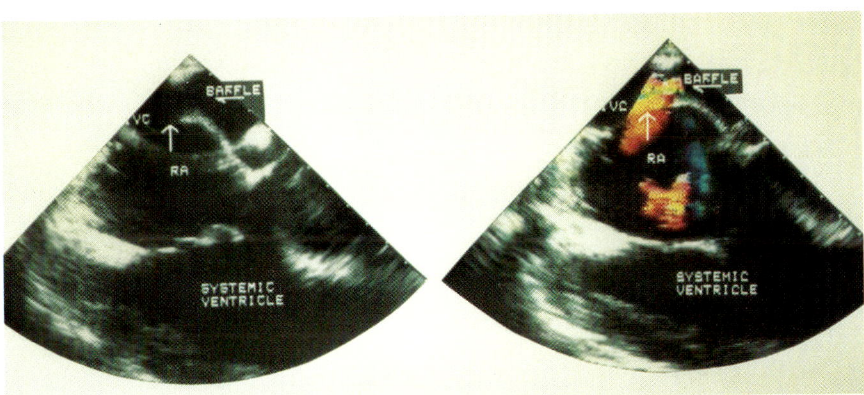

FIGURE 11-12. Imaging in the lower esophagus of the inferior limb of a Mustard baffle. There is a novel ventricular septum (VS) communication between the inferior vena cava and the right atrium (*arrow*), indicating breakdown of the baffle at this point.

At cardiac catheterization, TEE findings of obstruction were confirmed in all cases. Two cases of baffle leak were missed by angiography, and multiple baffle leaks in two cases could not be identified. Thus TEE appears to allow more detailed insight into abnormal baffle morphology and its related hemodynamic abnormalities than either transthoracic echocardiography or cardiac catheterization.

Complex Congenital Heart Disease

In the diagnosis of complex congenital heart disease, identification of atrial situs is the first step in sequential chamber localization. Before the advent of TEE in clinical practice, determination of atrial situs was made by radiographic examination of bronchus morphology or examination of abdominal great vessel orientation. TEE allows direct identification of atrial appendage morphology and location and thus atrial situs. The morphologic right atrial appendage has a short blunt appearance and broad junction with the right atrial cavity, whereas the left atrial appendage has a long, narrow, and crenelated appearance and a narrow junction with the left atrial cavity. Using these features, Stumper et al. were able to identify atrial situs correctly in 125 consecutive TEE examinations. In a study of 58 children, Stumper et al. identified four with juxtaposition of the atrial appendages.

Other Disorders

Coarctation of the Aorta

TEE demonstrates discrete narrowing of the descending aorta at the site of coarctation. Biplane TEE may demonstrate this better than the single-plane probe. Surface echocardiography with continuous wave Doppler allows parallel interrogation of blood flow across the coarctation and measurement of the transstenotic gradient. TEE probes with continuous wave capabilities will probably not add substantially to the quantitation of this disorder. TEE has proved useful, however, for assessment of aortic morphology and identification of intimal aortic dissection flaps following balloon dilatation.

Ebstein's Anomaly

TEE allows better definition of the morphology and function of the septal and posterior tricuspid leaflet and identification of any associated anomalies (atrial septal defect) (Fig. 11-13).

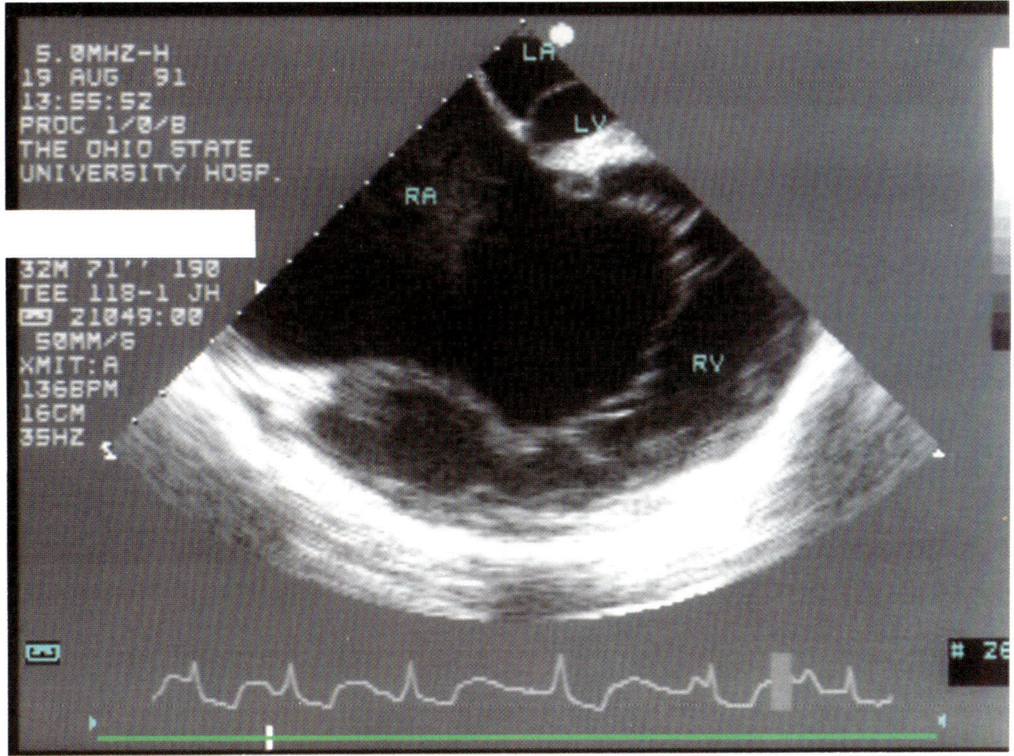

FIGURE 11-13. Transverse imaging of Ebstein's anomaly. The right atrium and right ventricle are massively dilated, and spontaneous contrast is noted in the right atrium. The abnormal tricuspid valve is noted with tethering along the right ventricular free wall.

Subaortic Membrane

TEE provides better definition of the morphology of the membrane and insertions into the mitral leaflet than does transthoracic echocardiography. Assessment of gradient is usually adequately made by transthoracic echocardiography.

Pulmonary Arteries

TEE allows better definition of the size and course of the main pulmonary artery, bifurcation, and proximal branch arteries. The pulmonary valve is better seen by surface echo. The right pulmonary artery can be visualized up to the crossing of the superior vena cava in most cases; thus peripheral pulmonary artery stenosis involving this branch is usually visualized. In contrast, with single-plane TEE, the left pulmonary artery is difficult to visualize beyond the bifurcation. Biplane TEE enhances imaging of the distal aspects of the pulmonary arteries.

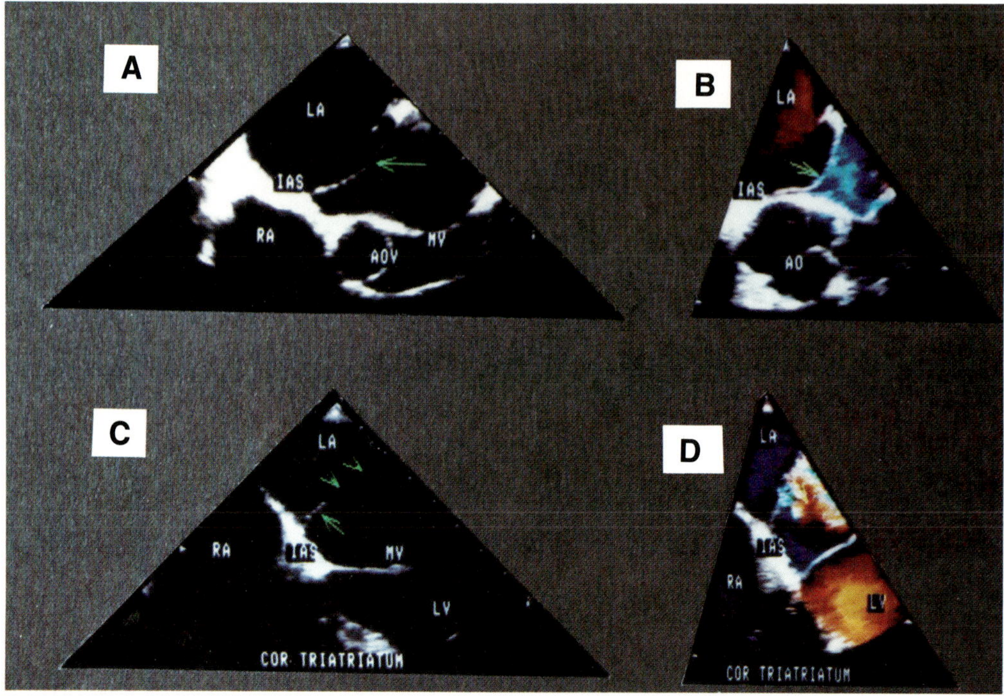

FIGURE 11-14. TEE images from patient with cor triatriatum. In the superior portion of the esophagus the membrane appears intact (A) with no color flow across it demonstrated (B). C. With advancement of the probe, a large hole in the membrane is identified (*arrowheads*). D. With color flow, high-velocity turbulence is identified.

Mitral Abnormalities

The anatomy of the mitral leaflets is usually well assessed by transthoracic echocardiography; however, in some situations, especially involving technically difficult transthoracic echocardiography, TEE may be indicated. In cleft mitral leaflet, an eccentric jet may be difficult to locate with surface echo, and TEE will usually add to the morphologic definition and more accurately assess mitral regurgitant severity with severely eccentric jets. We have also found TEE useful for differentiating congenital mitral abnormalities from possible vegetations caused by endocarditis (figure additional commissure, papillary muscle). Cor triatriatum TEE allows precise identification of attachment points of left atrium membrane and size of hole (Fig. 11-14).

Bicuspid Aortic Valve

TEE allows superior determination of aortic leaflet morphology (Fig. 11-15).

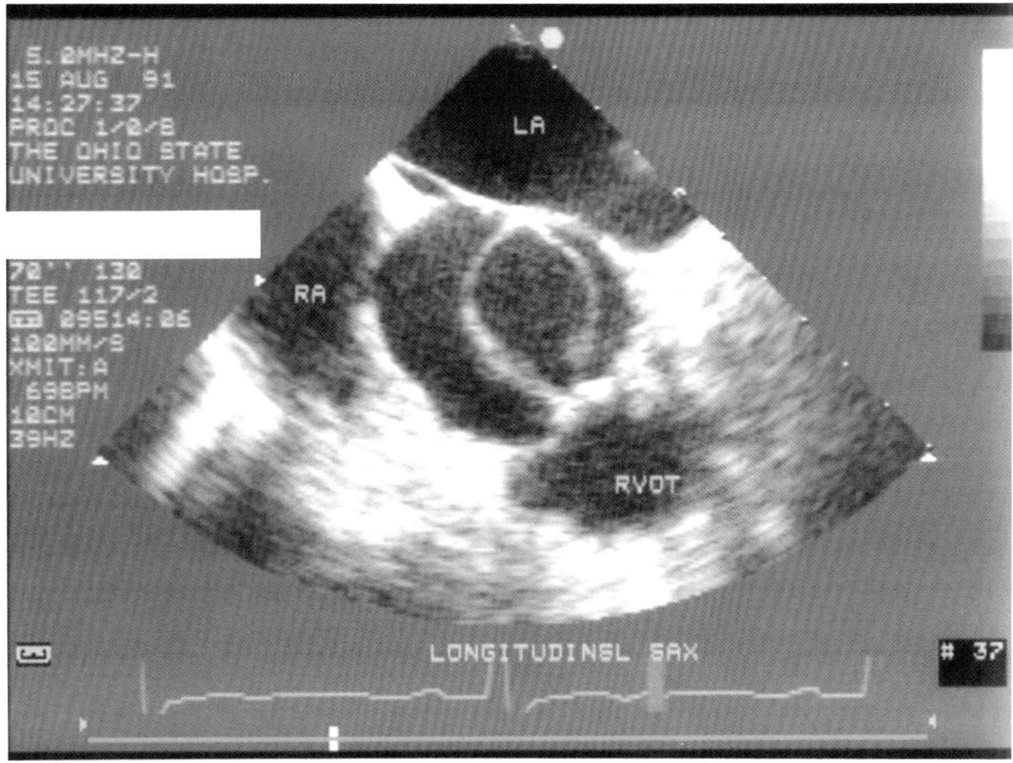

FIGURE 11-15. Bicuspid aortic valve with commissure line running from 11 o'clock to 5 o'clock. Longitudinal imaging with rightward motion of tip will usually allow imaging in the short axis to define aortic leaflet morphology better.

Patent Ductus

TEE is often helpful in the diagnosis of communications between the pulmonary artery and aorta. Both the location and direction of the shunt can be identified (Fig. 11-16).

TEE in Children

With the development of a special smaller (7 × 8 mm tip) TEE probe, experience with TEE in children with congenital heart disease is expanding. Stumper et al. examined 25 anesthetized children ranging in age from 1 year to 15 years and weight from 6.5 kg to 52 kg undergoing cardiac catheterization or intracardiac surgery. They found it useful in a more detailed evaluation of the morphology and function of the systemic and pulmonary venous return; the atrial, interatrial baffles; atri-

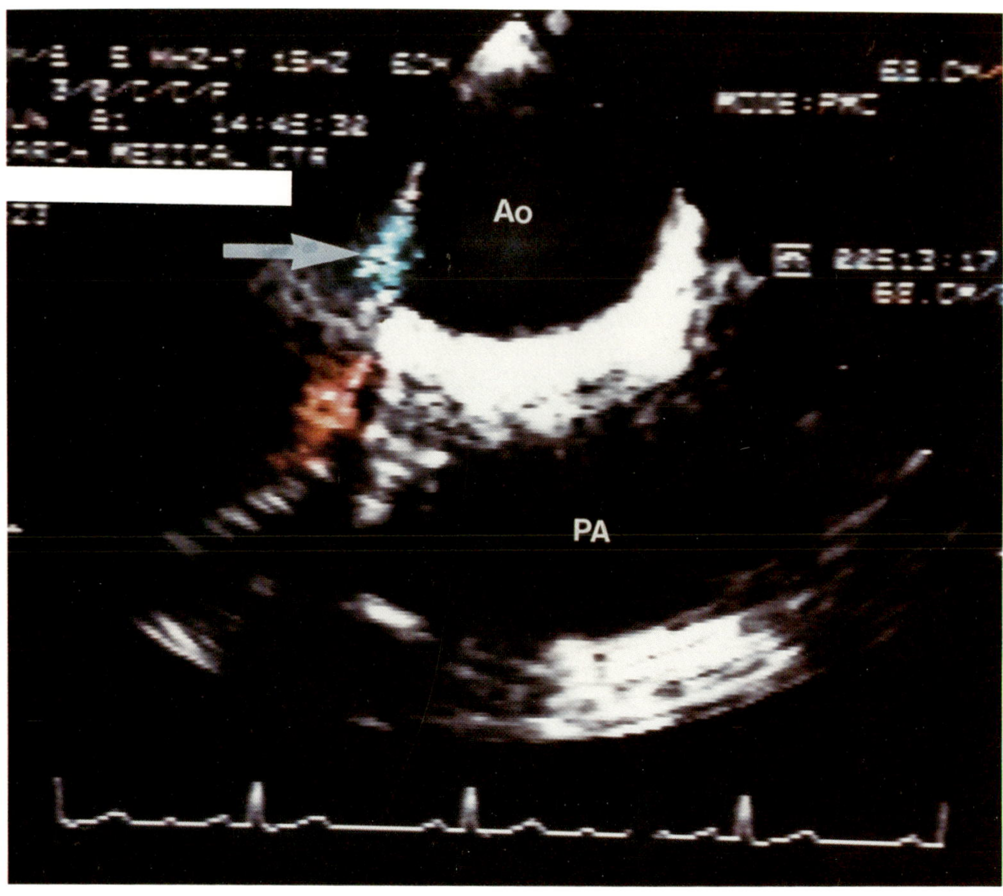

FIGURE 11-16. TEE image showing the communication (*arrow*) between the aorta (Ao) and pulmonary artery (PA) in a patient with a patent ductus.

oventricular valves; and left ventricular outflow tract, obtaining information in 60% of cases not obtainable by surface echocardiography. Use of TEE for intraoperative studies is becoming increasingly widespread.

Bibliography

Hanrath, P., Schluter, M., Langenstein, B.A., et al.: Detection of ostium secundum atrial septal defects by transesophageal cross-sectional echocardiography. Br. Heart J., 49:350–358, 1983.

Hellenbrand, W.E., Fahey, J.T., McGowan, F.X., et al.: Transesophageal echocardiographic guidance of transcatheter closure of atrial septal defect. Am. J. Cardiol., 66:207–213, 1990.

Huhta, J.C., Glasow, P., Murphy, D.J., et al.: Surgery without catheterization for congenital heart defects: Management of 100 patients. J. Am. Coll. Cardiol., 9:823, 1987.

Kaulitz, R., Stumper, O.F.W., Geusken, R., et al.: Comparative values of the precordial and transesophageal approaches in the echocardiographic evaluation of atrial baffle function after an atrial correction procedure. J. Am. Coll. Cardiol., 16(3):686–694, 1990.

Kronzon, I., Tunick, P.A., Freedberg, R.S., et al.: Transesophageal echocardiography is superior to transthoracic echocardiography in the diagnosis of sinus venosus atrial septal defect. J. Am. Coll. Cardiol., 17:537–542, 1991.

Morimoto, K., Matsuzake, M., Tohma, Y., et al.: Diagnosis and quantitative evaluation of secundum-type atrial septal defect by transesophageal Doppler echocardiography. Am. J. Cardiol., 66:85–91, 1990.

Shub, C., Dimopoulos, I.N., Seward, J.B., et al.: Sensitivity of two-dimensional echo in the direct visualization of atrial septal defect utilizing the subcostal approach: Experience with 154 patients. J. Am. Coll. Cardiol., 2:127, 1983.

Stumper, O.F.W., Elzenga, N.J., Hess, J., and Sutherland, G.R.: Transesophageal echocardiography in children with congenital heart disease: An initial experience. J. Am. Coll. Cardiol., 16(2):433–441, 1990.

Stumper, O.F.W., Fijlaarsdam, M., Vargas-Barron, J., et al.: The assessment of juxtaposed atrial appendages by transesophageal echocardiography. Int. J. Cardiol., 29:365–371, 1990.

Stumper, O.F.W., Sreeram, N., Elzenga, N.F., and Sutherland, G.R.: Diagnosis of atrial situs by transesophageal echocardiography. J. Am. Coll. Cardiol., 16(2):442–446, 1990.

12

Valvular Regurgitation

Over the past decade, standard transthoracic Doppler echocardiographic studies have become the noninvasive procedure of choice in the evaluation of patients with suspected or known valvular regurgitant lesions. In fact, studies using conventional Doppler echocardiography have reported sensitivities superior to auscultation in the evaluation of insufficient lesions and compare quite well to invasive assessment of the same. Owing to certain technical limitations, however, including acoustic impedance, evaluation of any individual patient using transthoracic echocardiography might be less than optimal. The transesophageal location of the transducer eliminates the problem of acoustic impedance in most patients and therefore provides an even more sensitive method in both the diagnosis and the quantitation of valvular insufficiency.

Mitral Regurgitation

Doppler echocardiography from the transesophageal window is an exquisitely sensitive technique in the diagnosis of mitral insufficiency (Fig. 12-1). The proximity of the left atrium to the transesophageal probe position and the absence of acoustic impedance allows an unimpeded view of the systolic mitral regurgitant jet. As in transthoracic studies, the maximal regurgitant color flow jet area seen with TEE correlates well with the degree of insufficiency (Fig. 12-2). The left atrium is evaluated in multiple planes to appreciate best the extent of the regurgitant jet. This is often accomplished by evaluating the left atrium in the four-chamber view and slowly flexing or withdrawing the probe to the basal short-axis level. Additionally the jet may be further interrogated while withdrawing the probe from the transgastric short-axis level through the mitral valve plane. Recent introduction of biplane transesophageal imaging techniques has added the capability of ex-

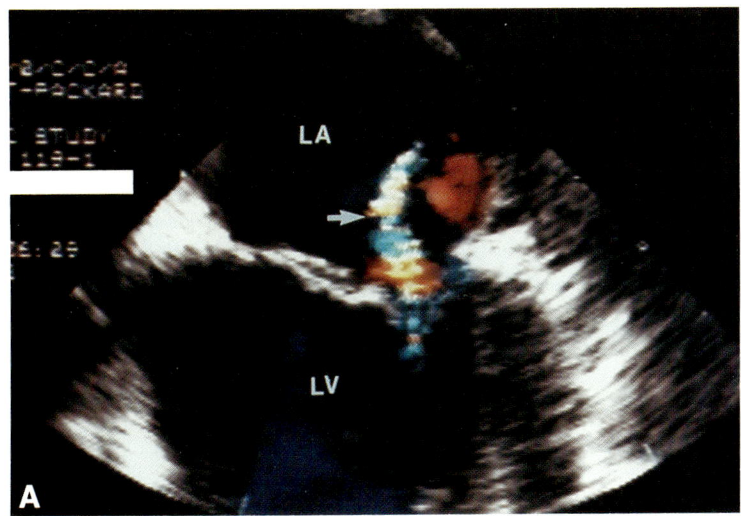

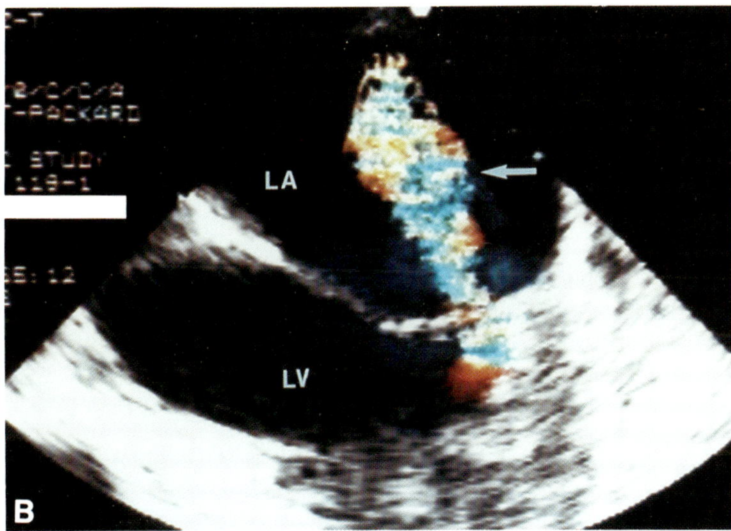

FIGURE 12-1. TEE images of patients with (A) mild and (B) moderate degrees of mitral insufficiency. Note the high-velocity mosaic jet (*arrow*) moving from the left ventricle (LV) into the left atrium (LA) during systole.

amining the mitral regurgitant jet in additional orthogonal planes, including both long-axis and two-chamber views.

Mitral regurgitation may occur secondary to a variety of causes. TEE imaging is extremely helpful in defining the etiology underlying the regurgitant lesion. The presence of a mitral valve vegetation, flail mitral valve leaflet, mitral valve prolapse, torn chordae, or papillary muscle rupture can each be diagnosed with accuracy by this technique.

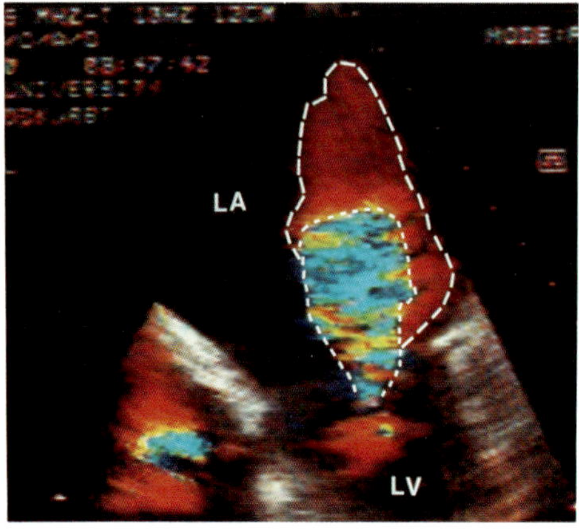

FIGURE 12-2. When estimating the maximal regurgitant jet area, it is important to measure only the mosaic high-velocity regurgitant jet (*small dashed line*) and not to include the low-velocity displaced blood as well.

Comparative Studies

TEE diagnosis and quantitation of mitral insufficiency have been compared with standard transthoracic Doppler echocardiography as well as left ventriculography. TEE appears to be significantly more sensitive in the diagnosis of mitral insufficiency. It has been shown that up to 30% of patients diagnosed with mitral regurgitation by TEE will have no evidence of mitral insufficiency by transthoracic study. Although the vast majority of these regurgitant jets will be of the mild variety, it is not rare that a moderate degree of insufficiency found on TEE will not be evident by transthoracic echocardiography. In a study of 138 patients by both TEE and transthoracic echocardiography, we have shown that there is agreement as to the grade of mitral regurgitation in only about 66% (Fig. 12-3). Factors including poor technical quality of transthoracic echocardiography and the presence of pros-

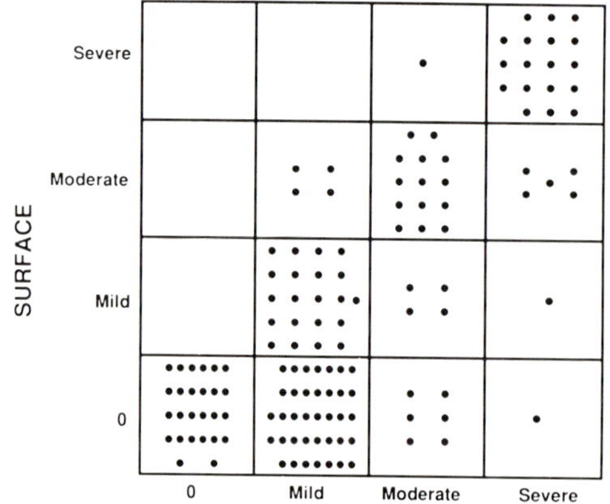

FIGURE 12-3. Comparison of transthoracic echocardiography (surface) and TEE in the diagnosis of mitral regurgitation ($n = 138$).

thetic heart valves precluding a complete evaluation of the left atrium limit the accuracy of transthoracic echo. Furthermore unobstructed imaging of the left atrium by TEE more often results in a larger mitral regurgitant jet area seen by this technique than by conventional transthoracic examination.

Likewise, TEE will frequently detect mild mitral insufficiency in patients in whom left ventriculography fails to reveal mitral regurgitation. Aside from these trivial degrees of mitral insufficiency, good correlation exists in the quantitation of mitral insufficiency by TEE and left ventriculography. We studied 48 patients undergoing TEE and left ventriculography. In general, the larger the maximal mitral regurgitant jet by TEE, the more significant the degree of mitral insufficiency found at left ventriculography. Absolute mitral regurgitant jet areas of less than 3 cm^2 correlated to mild angiographic insufficiency, from 3 to 6 cm^2 with moderate angiographic insufficiency, and greater than 6 cm^2 with severe angiographic insufficiency (Fig. 12-4). Patients with a flail mitral valve leaflet and a markedly eccentric jet might have a smaller regurgitant jet for their respective degree of insufficiency. This probably results from the loss of energy on impact of the regurgitant jet along the atrial wall (Fig. 12-5). Evaluation of pulmonary venous flow may be helpful in assessing the degree of insufficiency in these patients.

Pulmonary Venous Flow

Evaluation of pulmonary venous flow by TEE has been shown to be a valuable adjunct in the quantitation of mitral insufficiency. Changes in loading conditions and left ventricular performance, particularly in the operating room, as well as eccentric regurgitant jets, secondary to flail mitral valve leaflets, have a potential to cause inaccurate assessment as to the degree of mitral insufficiency. Pulmonary venous flow can be easily interrogated by transesophageal Doppler echocardiography (Fig. 12-6). In the normal individual, antegrade flow from the pulmonary vein into the left atrium is usually represented by biphasic systolic and diastolic forward components with a brief period of flow

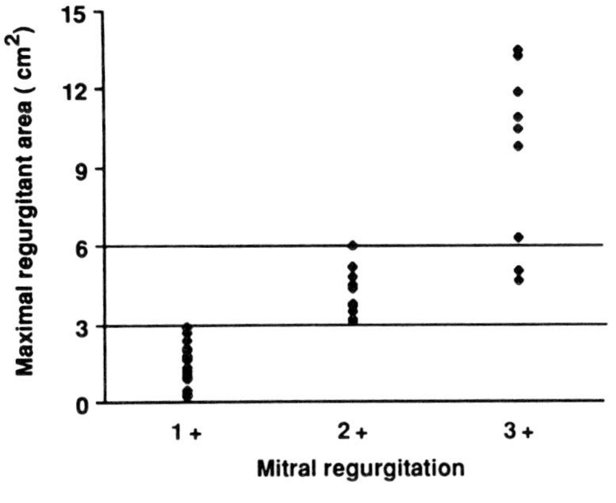

FIGURE 12-4. Comparison of the maximal regurgitant jet area as measured by TEE and 1 − 3+ mitral insufficiency at left ventriculography. Note that regurgitant jet areas of less than 3 cm^2 and areas greater than 6 cm^2 corresponded to mild and severe insufficiency, respectively.

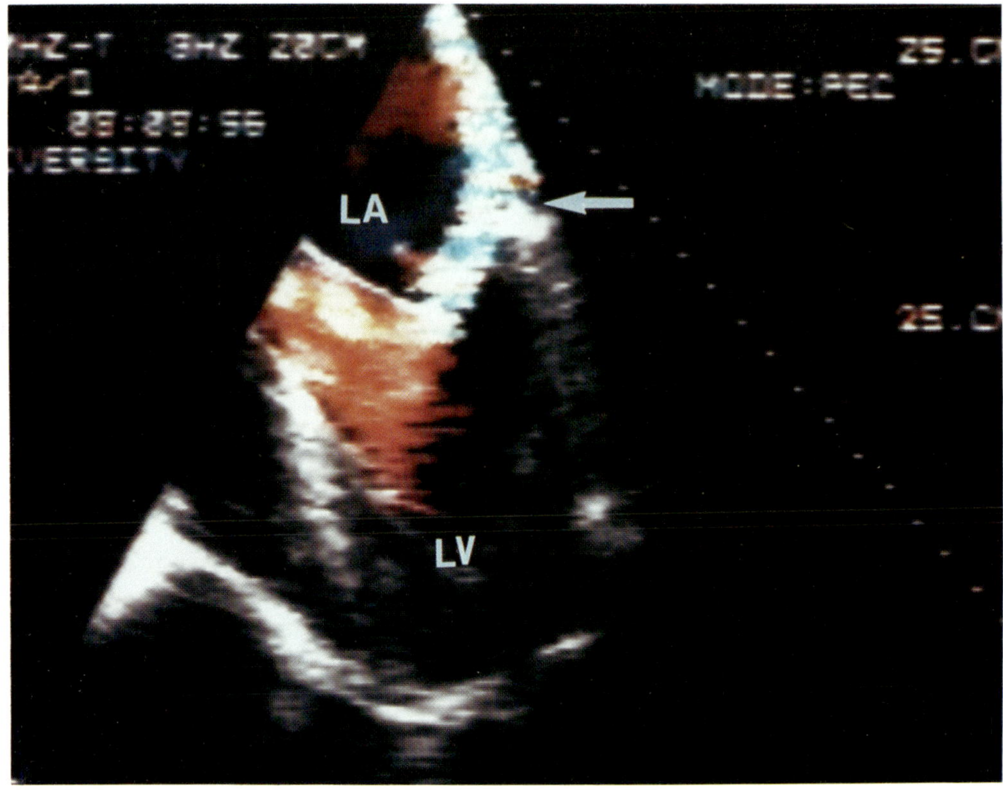

FIGURE 12-5. Posteriorly directed regurgitant jet from patient with flail anterior mitral valve leaflet.

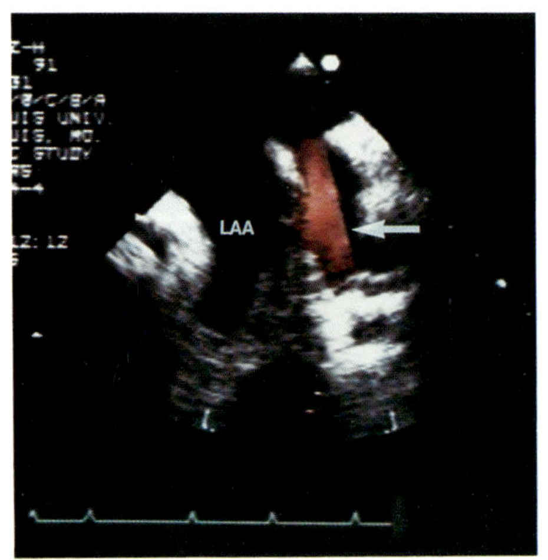

FIGURE 12-6. The left upper pulmonary vein can usually be visualized and pulmonary venous flow sampled from the upper esophagus.

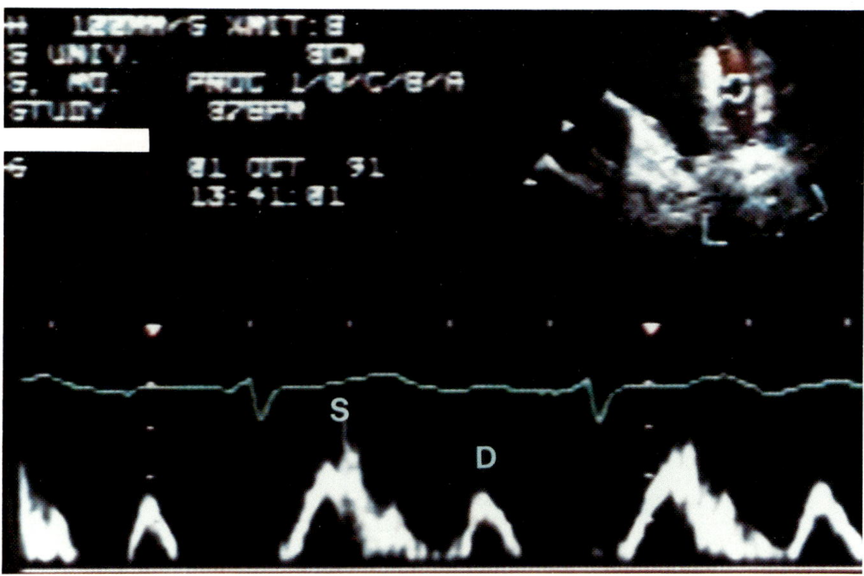

FIGURE 12-7. Normal pulmonary venous flow demonstrating the systolic (S), diastolic (D) and (A) wave 2 degrees to atrial systole.

reversal corresponding to atrial systole (Fig. 12-7). Patients with significant mitral insufficiency will often have a blunted or reversed systolic component to their pulmonary venous flow (Fig. 12-8). This additional information should be obtained and used when quantitating the degree of mitral insufficiency by TEE (Fig. 12-9).

Aortic Insufficiency

TEE is a useful technique in the evaluation of patients with suspected aortic insufficiency. Turbulent diastolic flow reversal can be appreciated from a basal short-axis view of the aorta (Fig. 12-10) or in the left ventricular outflow tract in the four-chamber or five-chamber view (Fig. 12-11). Addition of biplane TEE capabilities allows a longitudinal or long-axis view of the left ventricular outflow tract and ascending aorta (Fig. 12-12), as well. Aortic insufficiency is most often graded according to the ratio of the regurgitant diastolic jet width and the left ventricular outflow tract diameter or the ratio of the regurgitant jet area to the aortic root area in the basal short-axis view. Several investigators have reported good results using the maximal regurgitant jet area as well. Imaging of the aortic valve leaflets and aortic root are greatly enhanced by the transesophageal position of the transducer. The relative lack of acoustic impedance allows better description of the aortic valve leaflets and thus a more accurate description of the cause of the regurgitant

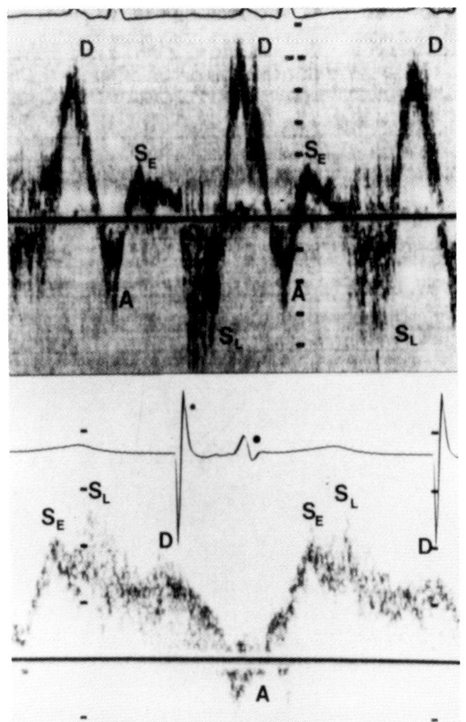

FIGURE 12-8. Preoperative (upper panel) and postoperative (lower panel) pulmonary venous flow recording in a patient undergoing mitral valve repair for significant mitral regurgitation at the marked flow reversal during late systole (S_L) seen preoperatively.

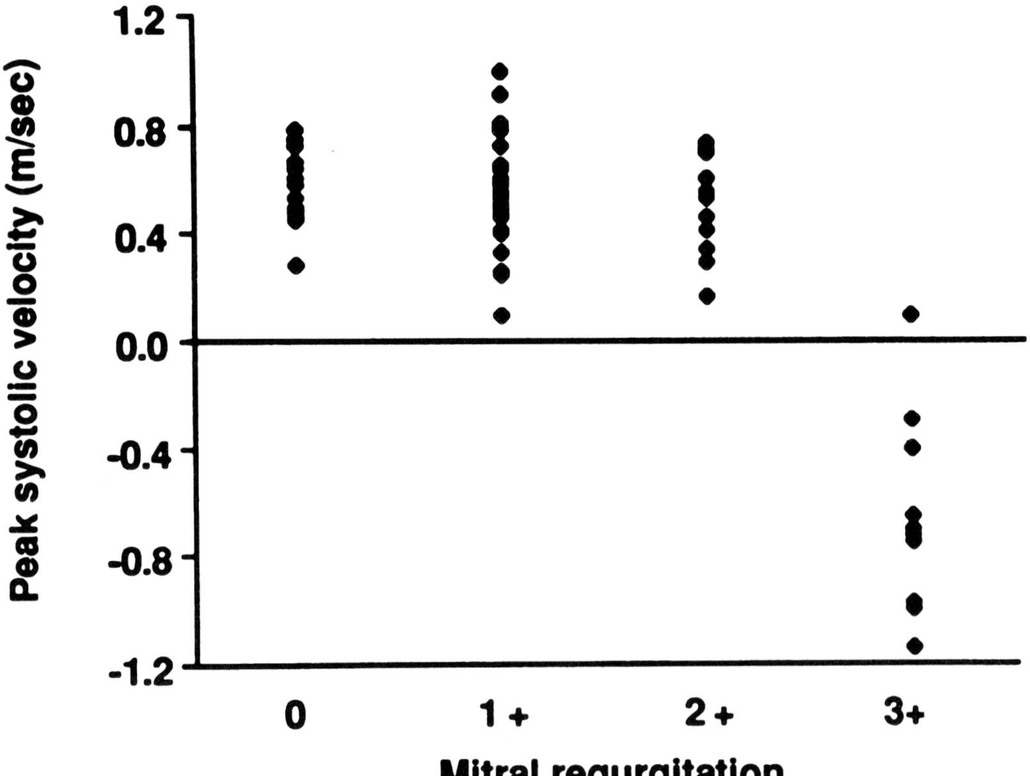

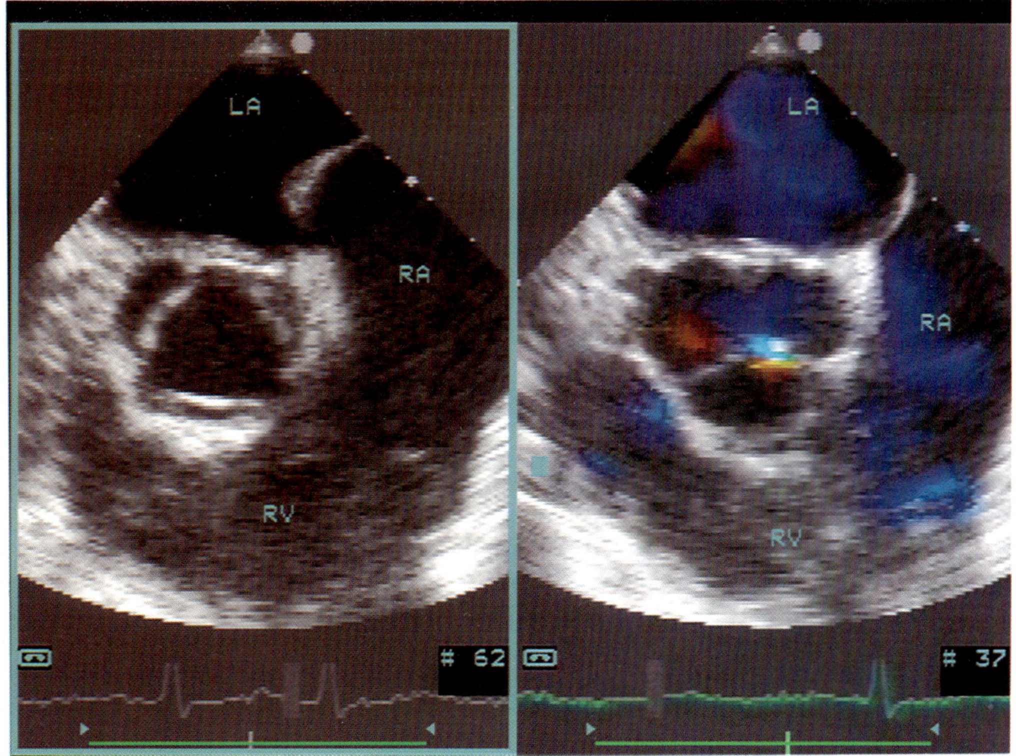

FIGURE 12-10. Systolic (left) and diastolic (right) basal short-axis images in a patient with mild aortic insufficiency. Note the minimal turbulent insufficient jet seen in the center of the aortic valve leaflets.

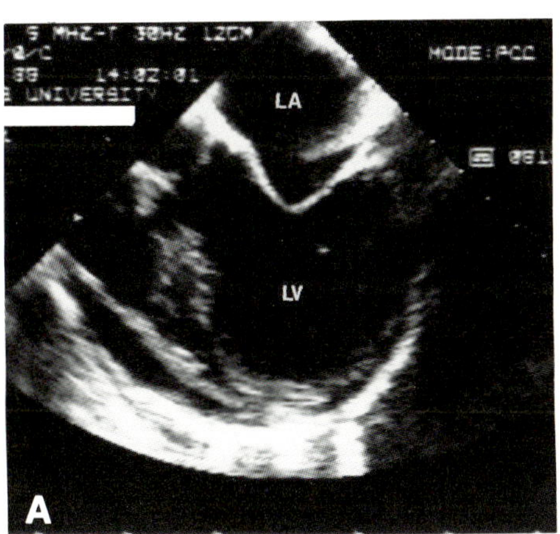

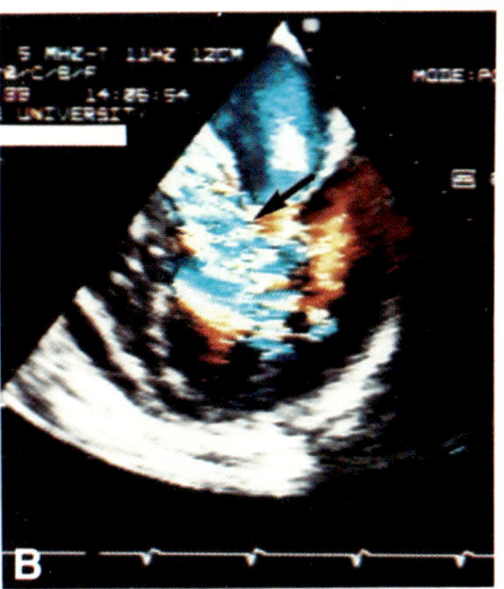

FIGURE 12-11. A and B. Two-dimensional echocardiographic five-chamber view in a patient with severe aortic insufficiency. Note how the insufficient jet (*arrow*) fills the left ventricular outflow tract with the color-flow turned on (B).

FIGURE 12-9. Relationship of the peak of forward systolic velocity in the left upper pulmonary vein in patients with 0 − 3+ mitral insufficiency. Note that patients with severe mitral regurgitation will have markedly blunted or reversed pulmonary venous systolic flow. (From Castello, R., Pearson, A.C., Lenzen, P., and Labovitz, A.J.: Effect of mitral regurgitation on pulmonary venous velocities derived from transesophageal echocardiography color-guided pulsed Doppler. J. Am. Coll. Cardiol., *17*:1499–1506, 1991.)

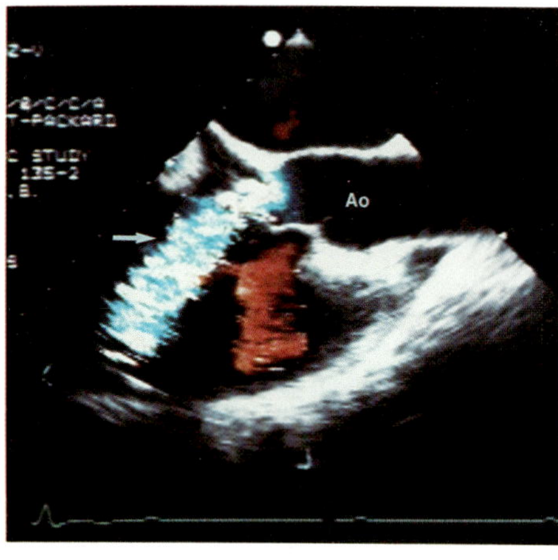

FIGURE 12-12. Longitudinal view of ascending aorta (Ao) in patient with significant aortic insufficiency A+ (*arrow*).

lesion. Calcific aortic valve disease, dilated aortic root, aortic valve endocarditis and proximal aortic dissection are all diagnosed with greater accuracy by TEE.

Comparative Studies

TEE appears to be slightly more sensitive than transthoracic echocardiography in the diagnosis of aortic insufficiency. It has been reported that up to 20% of those patients diagnosed with aortic insufficiency by TEE will have negative studies by transthoracic echocardiography. In general, these patients include only those with mild degrees of aortic insufficiency. Conversely transthoracic echocardiography occasionally will reveal the presence of aortic insufficiency not appreciated by TEE. This occurs primarily in patients with calcified aortic valves in whom the regurgitant jet is either shadowed

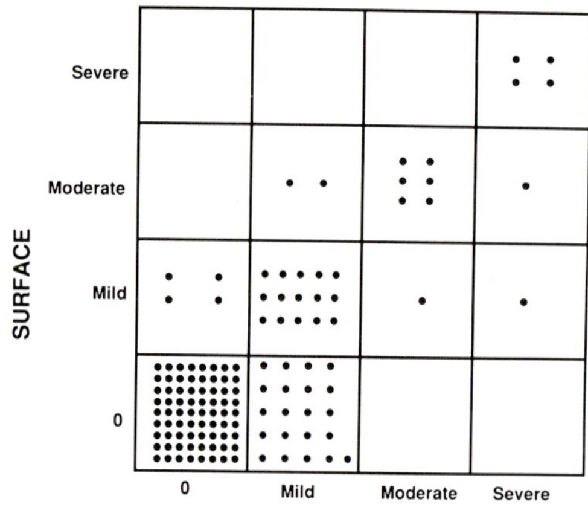

FIGURE 12-13. Comparison of transthoracic (surface) and transesophageal echo in the diagnosis and quantitation of aortic regurgitation ($n = 118$).

or occurs as an eccentric angle secondary to dilatation of the root. In a study of 118 patients undergoing both TEE and transthoracic echocardiography, we found agreement between the two techniques of about 85% (Fig. 12-13). In general, the size of aortic regurgitant jets is greater when seen by TEE compared with transthoracic study. Biplane technique should enhance the diagnostic sensitivity of TEE in patients with aortic insufficiency.

Tricuspid and Pulmonic Insufficiency

Both tricuspid and pulmonic insufficiency are noted with great frequency by transthoracic echocardiography even in the normal individual. TEE is probably no more sensitive than transthoracic echocardiography in the diagnosis of right-sided valvular regurgitation except in the technically difficult patient. TEE may, however, allow the diagnosis of associated abnormalities, particularly when there is right atrial pathology present.

Bibliography

Castello, R.: Comparison of transesophageal echocardiography/cath. J. Am. Coll. Cardiol. (in press).

Castello, R., Fagan, L., Lenzen, P., et al.: Comparison of transthoracic and transesophageal echocardiography for assessment of left-sided valvular regurgitation. Am. J. Cardiol. (in press).

Castello, R., Pearson, A.C., Lenzen, P., and Labovitz, A.J.: Effect of mitral regurgitation on pulmonary venous velocities derived from transesophageal echocardiography color-guided pulsed Doppler. J. Am. Coll. Cardiol., 17:1499–1506, 1991.

Kleinman, J.P., Czer, L.S.C., DeRobertis, M., et al.: A quantitative comparison of transesophageal and epicardial color Doppler echocardiography in the intraoperative assessment of mitral regurgitation. Am. J. Cardiol., 64:1168–1172, 1989.

Smith, M.D., Harrison, M.R., Pinton, R., et al.: Regurgitant jet size by transesophageal compared with transthoracic Doppler color flow imaging. Circulation, 83:79–86, 1991.

Yoshida, K., Yoshikawa, J., Yamaura, Y., et al.: Assessment of mitral regurgitation by biplane transesophageal color Doppler flow mapping. Circulation, 82:1121–1126, 1990.

13

Valvular Stenosis

Aortic Stenosis

Surface echocardiography can usually identify quite accurately anatomic abnormalities of the aortic valve. As such, the cause of aortic stenosis, that is, calcific degenerative changes, bicuspid aortic valve, or rheumatic pathology, can usually be ascertained by careful examination. Some idea of the hemodynamic severity of aortic stenosis can be gained by observing the orifice or opening of the valve during systole. These observations are usually not useful for clinical decision making, however, and until the advent of continuous wave Doppler echocardiography, the severity of aortic stenosis was almost always confirmed by cardiac catheterization.

From transthoracic windows using continuous wave Doppler, the highest transaortic velocities can be recorded. The peak and mean pressure gradient across the valve can then be determined by application of the Bernoulli equation. Accurate surface Doppler examinations require meticulous attention to recording quality, with acquisition of flow signals from multiple sites, including apex, suprasternal notch, and right parasternal window, to ensure near-parallel interrogation. Accurate determination of aortic valve area by the continuity equation is made by acquiring pulsed Doppler recordings of left ventricular outflow tract velocity and measuring the diameter of the left ventricular outflow tract. The percentage of technically unsatisfactory studies for aortic stenosis is low in our experience (<5%) even in patients with poor two-dimensional images.

TEE may be useful in some circumstances in the assessment of aortic stenosis. The improved visualization of the aortic valve afforded by the esophageal window and higher frequency, near field imaging appears to make planimetry of the stenotic orifice more accurate than by transthoracic echocardiography. Thus in the patient with technically difficult transthoracic examinations, the basal short-axis scan at the level of the aortic leaflets from TEE can give an estimate of the severity of aortic stenosis. In measurement of the aortic valve area, it is important to obtain true short-axis views of the aortic leaflets. Satisfactory images are recognized by the circular appearance of the aorta and usually require forward flexion of the scope tip 70 to 90 degrees along with leftward flexion to 70 to 90 degrees. With TEE probes having biplane imaging capabilities, the probe tip in the longitudinal plane is flexed slightly rightward and forward to obtain short-axis images. Imaging of the aortic valve orifice is optimized by slight advancement or withdrawal of the probe to visualize the aortic leaflet cusps. Gain settings are minimized. The valve orifice area is traced as the innermost edges of the aortic valve cusps at maximal systolic separation (Figs. 13-1 and 13-2). Planimetry of the visualized orifice using these techniques has correlated well with known cardiac catheterization–derived valve areas and those obtained by the continuity equation from surface echocardiography.

Technical limitations to this measurement, however, should be kept in mind. First, in some patients as a result of tortuosity of the ascending aorta, a true short-axis scan of the aortic leaflets is not possible. Thus overestimation or underestimation of the valve area may occur. Biplane imaging, in our experience, almost always allows this true short-axis

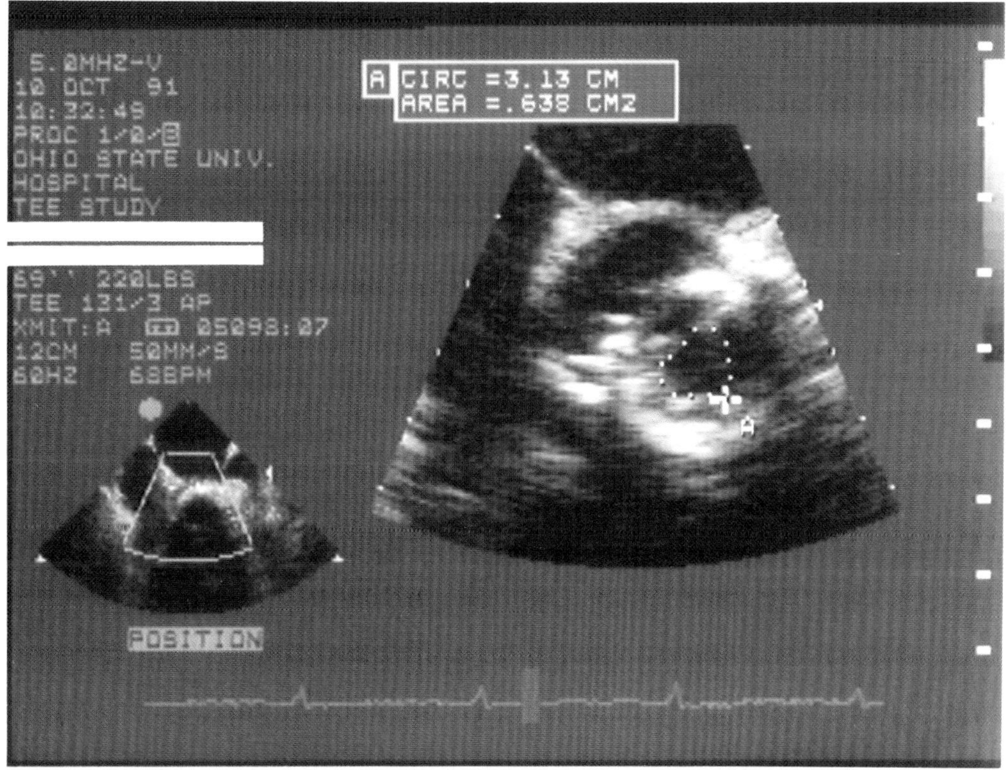

FIGURE 13-1. Planimetry of valve area of 12-year-old porcine aortic prosthesis. The valve area of 0.75 cm^2 agreed well with catheter-derived (0.9 cm^2) and Doppler-derived (0.9 cm^2) areas.

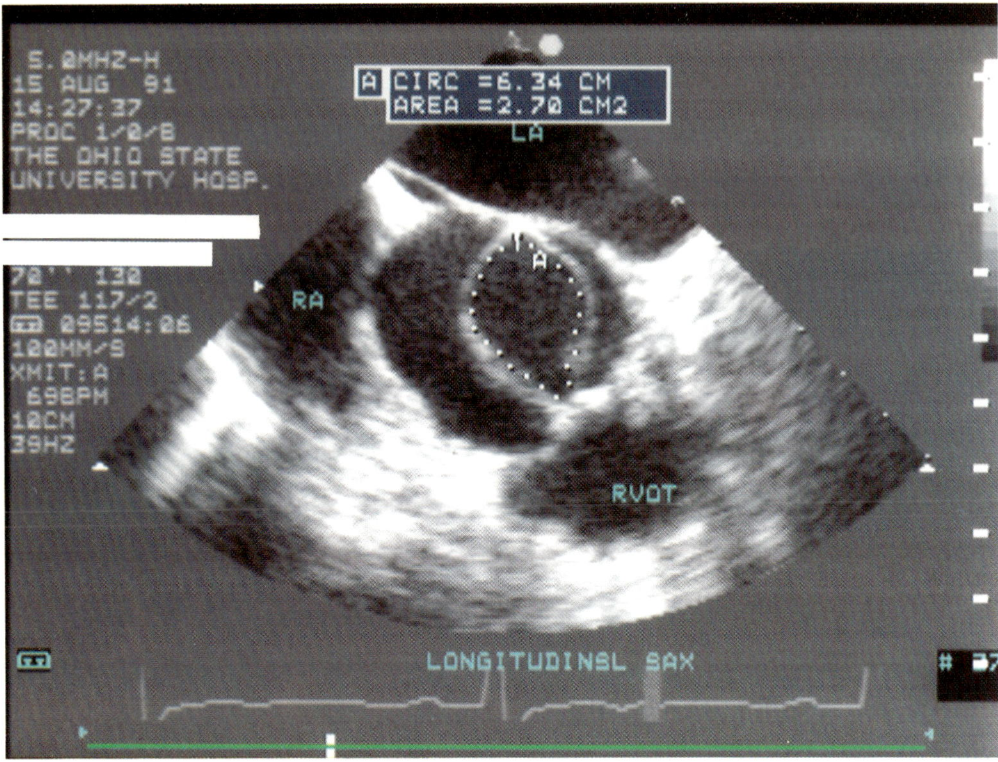

FIGURE 13-2. Planimetry of native bicuspid aortic valve.

scan to be obtained. Second, in heavily calcified valves, blooming of echoes may artificially reduce the true flow area. Third, in low flow states, the valve leaflets may not open to the fullest extent allowable because of reduced driving pressures.

Despite these caveats, this measurement may prove useful in certain circumstances. First, intraoperatively, following an aortic valve repair or debridement, a quick assessment of valve orifice can be obtained by TEE using this technique. Second, in the patient in whom surface echocardiography is so poor that adequate continuous wave recordings of the peak aortic velocities are not obtainable (these are rare in our experience), a TEE may be considered to obtain valve area.

With more and more probes being outfitted with continuous wave Doppler, there is hope that TEE will be able to assess accurately the hemodynamics of aortic stenosis (Fig. 13-3). The major drawback of single-plane TEE in this regard has been the inability to obtain multiple interrogation windows on the aortic valve to insure parallel interrogation of the aortic stenosis jet. Thus preliminary reports have indicated that TEE continuous wave interrogation of aortic stenosis tends to underestimate the valve gradient and overestimate the valve areas. With

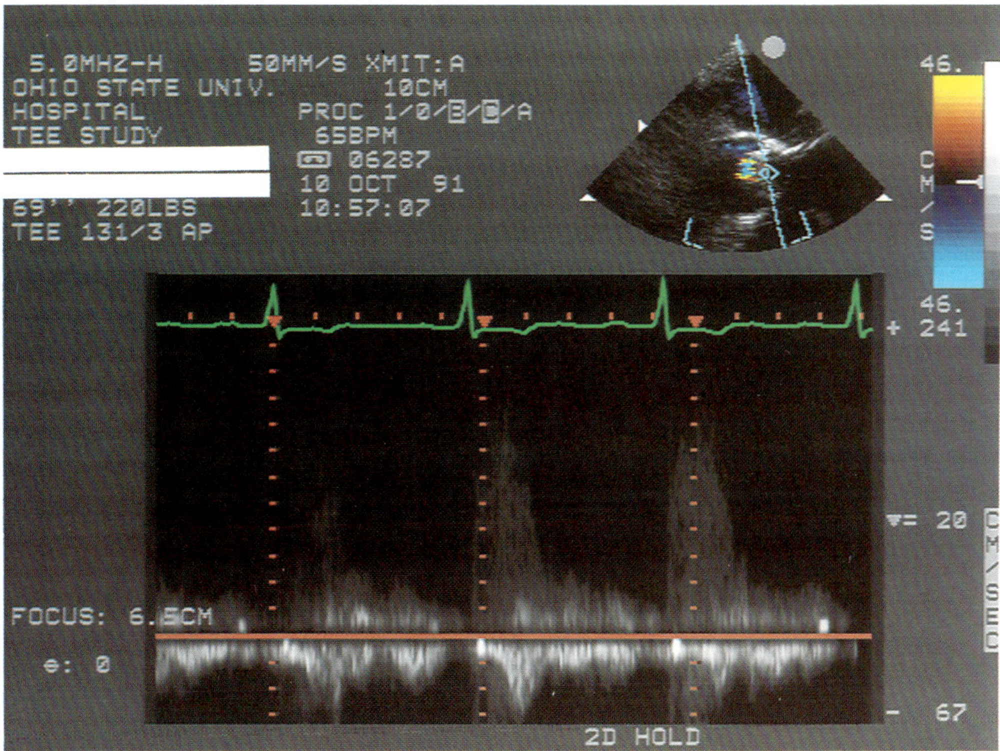

FIGURE 13-3. Continuous wave recordings from stenotic aortic valve.

continuous wave Doppler combined with biplane imaging, this limitation is somewhat overcome. Until more confirmation of the accuracy of TEE with continuous wave Doppler in aortic stenosis, however, greater reliance should be placed on either imaging of the aortic valve area or transthoracic echocardiographic continuous wave recordings. The width of the color flow jet as it crosses the stenosed aortic valve has also been used as a measure of the severity of aortic stenosis (Fig. 13-4).

Mitral Stenosis

Precordial two-dimensional echocardiographic imaging of the stenotic mitral valve orifice is considered by many to be the gold standard in the assessment of mitral stenosis because the anatomic orifice is not influenced by the presence of mitral regurgitation, cardiac output, and other factors that influence catheterization-determined valve areas. Ac-

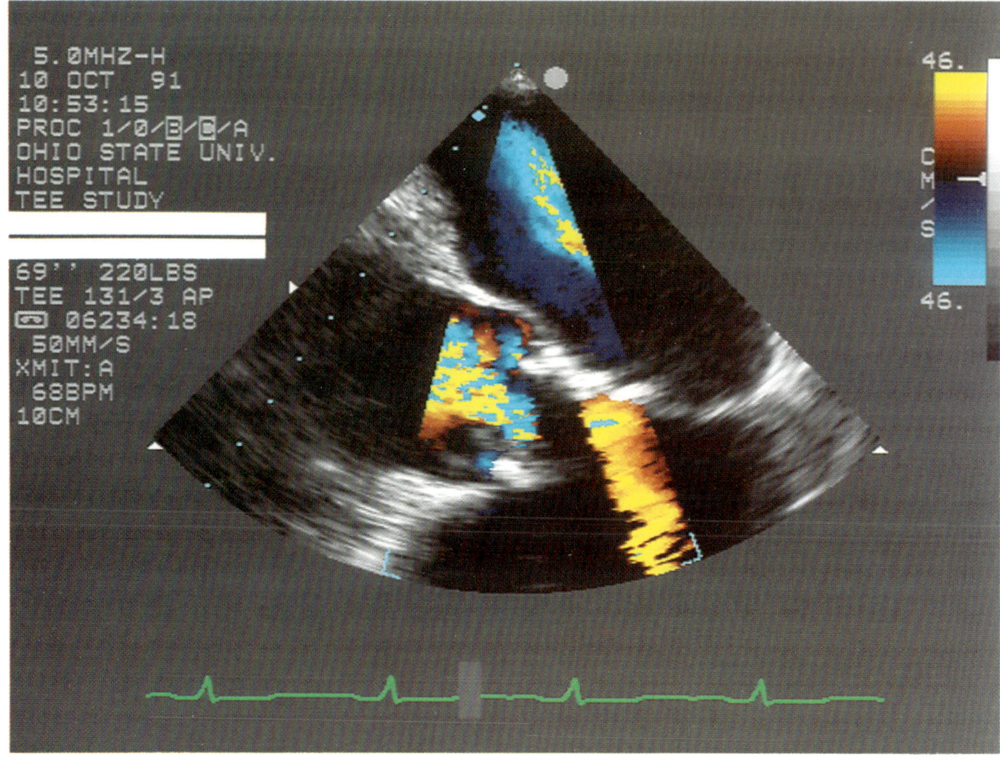

FIGURE 13-4. Color flow recording of aortic stenosis.

curate measurement, however, requires considerable expertise and meticulous attention to technique.

Doppler echocardiography can be used to measure the velocities across the stenotic mitral valve. When significant mitral stenosis is present, higher velocities reflect accurately the elevated left atrial/left ventricular pressure gradient. The gradient can be calculated by planimetry of the velocities and use of the Bernoulli equation. The pressure half-time technique quantitates the rate at which the left atrial/left ventricular pressure gradient decays in early diastole and allows a relatively accurate method for determination of mitral valve area. Factors other than valve area clearly influence pressure half-time, however, including left atrial and ventricular compliance, initial pressure gradient, and aortic insufficiency.

Although excellent short-axis images of the mitral valve can be obtained by TEE in many cases, there are no data to suggest that planimetry of the valve accurately reflects valve area. In our experience, in fact, a consistent overestimate of the stenotic orifice occurs from TEE short-axis planes. The reasons for this have not been elucidated, but a major difficulty may be insuring a true short-axis cut. In addition, visualization of the effective flow-limiting orifice can be problematic.

Combination imaging/continuous wave TEE single-plane probes have demonstrated that the mitral pressure gradient and pressure half-time can be accurately measured by TEE. Flow through the mitral valve, in contrast to that through the aortic valve, is almost always within 30 degrees of parallel to the ultrasound beam during TEE examination. Thus gradients are unlikely to be underestimated. The incremental value of the TEE quantitation of mitral stenosis has yet to be fully determined. Evaluation of these patients for assessment of valve calcification and mobility as well as associated regurgitation, however, may be helpful in selecting appropriate candidates for balloon valvuloplasty.

Bibliography

Hofmann, T., Kasper, W., Meinertz, T., et al.: Determination of aortic valve orifice area in aortic valve stenosis by two-dimensional transesophageal echocardiography. Am. J. Cardiol., 59:330–335, 1987.

Index

Note: Page numbers in *italics* indicate figures; t indicates tables